ALLERGY-PROOF RECIPES for KIDS

More Than 150 Recipes That Are All Wheat-Free, Gluten-Free, Nut-Free, Egg-Free, Dairy-Free, and Low in Sugar

LESLIE HAMMOND and **LYNNE MARIE ROMINGER**

Foreword by Kevin A. Tracy, M.D., Specialist in
Pediatric Internal Medicine at the UC Davis Medical Group

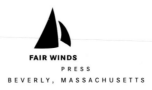

FAIR WINDS
PRESS
BEVERLY, MASSACHUSETTS

First published in the USA in 2003 by
Fair Winds Press, a member of
Quayside Publishing Group
100 Cummings Center, Suite 406-L
Beverly, MA 01915
www.fairwindspress.com

Library of Congress Cataloging-in-Publication Data available

ISBN-13: 978-1-59233-383-7
ISBN-10: 1-59233-383-4

15 14 13 12 10   3 4 5

Cover design by Kathie Alexander
Book design by Kathie Alexander

Printed and bound in China

The information in this book is for educational purposes only. It is not intended to
replace the advice of a physician or medical practitioner. Please see your health
care provider before beginning any new health program.

Dedication

All "free-food" kids—regardless of an allergy, disease, intolerance, or choice, here is something yummy for you!

For my Grandpa John and Grandma Jenny
— Leslie Hammond

For my mother
— Lynne Marie Rominger

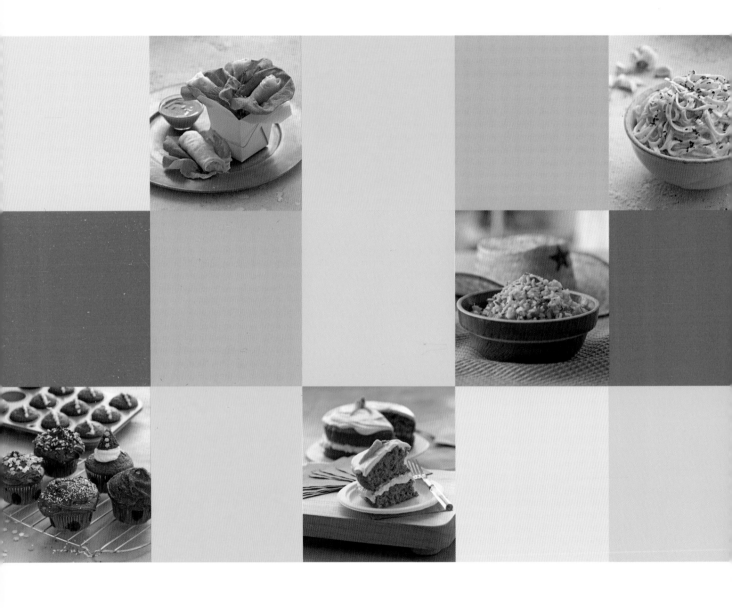

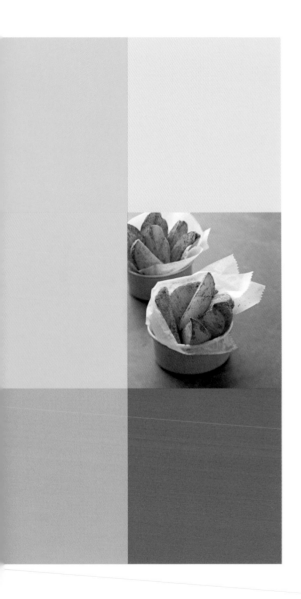

Table of Contents

Foreword

"What's for dinner?" "Is there anything to eat?" "Can I have some of that?" Not a day goes by that thoughts of food do not enter our minds, pushing aside whatever else is in there when we are hungry. Moreover, we eat if we are happy; we eat if we are sad. We celebrate big events and those smaller special moments with food. We socialize over brunch, meet family for lunch, and get together with old friends for dinner. In times of trouble, eating comforts us. And what would holidays and birthdays, weddings, and graduations be like without their associated feasts, potlucks, and special dishes? Take away the social nature of our food and there most certainly would be a revolution. Like water and shelter, we need food to live. Humans need food on many levels—of course physiological but also emotional!

So what happens when food—that which we desire, crave, and need— makes us ill? Food intolerances and allergies can cause everything from chronic aches and pains to life-threatening reactions. Identifying and avoiding offending foods may be simple or it may drastically alter your life. It's not easy for adults to stay clear of whatever foods may harm them; it's even more difficult for children.

What does a child with a food allergy do at a birthday party, at school, or at a friend's house when something wonderful is served that contains something "bad"? Saying "no, thank you" when everyone else is gobbling up the delicious treat is hard to do. Should you just try a little, so no one will think you are contrary or weird, risking turning red with hives and stopping breathing or suffering with stomachaches for days? Such are the dilemmas faced by those trying to eat the right thing.

As a pediatrician, I see many parents who believe their child's various complaints and problems are due to food allergies. Most are not, and when there are specific food interactions, they are usually not true allergies but are common reactions and intolerances. Even so, some parents become afraid to feed their infants or children for fear of what may happen. But then there are those children who suffer with true food allergies, which make their eczema and asthma worse, may cause poor growth, can cause horrible intestinal problems, or can suddenly bring about severe breathing trouble. Daily life can prove simple or hard, depending upon how easy it is to eliminate and avoid the offending food and how cooperative the child is at following the food rules. Unfortunately, that which is forbidden quickly becomes more attractive. Moreover, others that are unaware the offered food is a no-no and potentially life-threatening for the child may give gifts, treats, and free samples.

One food that causes allergic reactions in many, wheat, is often called the "staff of life." But wheat can be the "disrupter of sleep" and "spoiler of play" for those with wheat and gluten sensitivities and allergies—as it was for the author of this book, Leslie Hammond.

I met Leslie when she was a child, trying to figure out why she had such bad belly pains and so many gastrointestinal problems. No one could figure out what was wrong with Leslie. After a hospitalization, I tested Leslie for many possibilities before we figured out what was ailing her, why she suffered so much. Food—"the staff of life," in particular—was making Leslie sick. The cookies that she craved and the toast that she was eating because it was "bland" (she figured everything else would further upset her stomach) were actually the culprits. But what foods that kids eat don't have wheat? What could Leslie eat? Well, from the motivation of personal experience, she has been successful in finding ways to enjoy mealtime without suffering later. This cookbook is to help families faced with the challenge of feeding the kids when foods are forbidden.

Leslie proves food can still be fun and the centerpiece of life's parties— even when food allergies are an issue. She manages this feat by putting the "usual" ingredients back on the shelf and replacing them with others you may have never used or never thought you could use. Recipes may at first taste or look a tad different, but with a happy body comes a happy mind, and soon we have new foods to comfort the soul and to answer the eternal question, "Isn't there anything else to eat?" Feeding a child with food allergies can be challenging for parents. All kids want yummy "kid-standard" fare like macaroni and cheese and spaghetti. All kids want a chocolate chip cookie now and then! With this book, every child gets a cookie, thanks to Leslie.

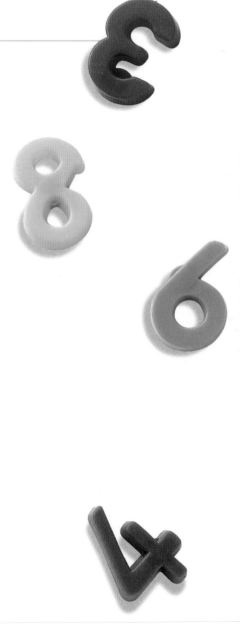

—**Kevin A. Tracy, MD**, Pediatric Internal Medicine, UC Davis Medical Group, Sacramento, California

Introduction

In a world full of sweets, treats, and fun foods like pizza, it's extremely difficult to be the child who is allergic to everything everyone else eats. So many menu items include wheat and dairy as staple ingredients—precisely the items that cause the most trouble for children and adults who suffer from food allergies. Think about what the favorite foods of most kids are. Perhaps pizza, spaghetti, chicken nuggets, and macaroni and cheese top the list. Now think about what their favorite sweets and treats are. Ask them, and most will include cookies, cupcakes, and brownies high on the list. And all those delights just mentioned—from the nuggets to the cupcakes—contain wheat flour and/or dairy elements. So what can a mom feed a hungry child who can't eat anything?

I have the answer because I was one of those children with food allergies. Until finally diagnosed with multiple food allergies, I endured a childhood beset by illness after illness. By my preteens, after a lengthy hospitalization, one doctor finally figured out why I was so sick all the time. But a diagnosis didn't end the heartache. In fact, my suffering was only beginning. I went home from the hospital to watch my siblings and parents eat everything delicious and appealing to the palate that I couldn't. On my thirteenth birthday, my friends and family sat down to a Baskin Robbins ice cream cake while I was handed a rice cracker! No wonder I hid bags of chocolate chip cookies in my closet and ate clandestinely, only to get sick again and again. The hard part I had to live with was being a normal person who felt abnormal because I had nothing to eat. If I ate what my friends and family ate, I would become sick. But even though I felt abnormal, I really wasn't that different because so many people suffer with food allergies. According to the National Institute of Allergy and Infectious Diseases, "food allergy occurs in 8 percent of children and in 1–2 percent of adults. Approximately 100 Americans, usually children, die annually from food-induced anaphylaxis." Currently, 5–8 million Americans (and statistics are on the rise) are allergic to a food. Strict avoidance of the restricted food is the only way to avoid a reaction, extreme illness, and in some cases, even death.

Recognizing the importance of avoiding wheat in my diet, I was determined to find a way to eat and enjoy delicious meals that wouldn't make me sick. So I started finding healthy substitutes and creating yummy foods that I could eat. When I started having children of my own (surprise: all with food allergies), I committed myself to finding ways to include the whole family in tasty repast and treats without any wheat and/or dairy. *Allergy-Proof Recipes for Kids* is built from my experience and includes realistic recipes for moms and dads of food-allergic families. All of my recipes are the types of dishes that you see kids eating at school, parties, and on the covers of magazines. Where once I was banned from eating pizza and cake on my birthday, I proudly show you parents how to make a pizza worthy of a trendy bistro and a Mock Hostess Cupcake one might find in a child's lunchbox. I've managed to offer bakery-style muffins instead of bland and funny-tasting foods to hungry, allergy-suffering mouths.

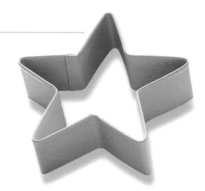

A goal of my cookbook is that you can walk into your local supermarket and purchase most of the ingredients you need to cook for your family—that you needn't travel to a specialty market to make dinner. Please refer to the shopping section of this cookbook for guidance.

Because I was hungry, I succeeded in making great-tasting common foods like pancakes and Hot and Yummy Pockets like the store brand, all allergy-free. Because I feel so adamantly that every child deserves to feel included at mealtime, I've gathered my recipes for your family in this cookbook. You can buy or make foods for the whole family that taste wonderful. Your child will love being part of the communal enjoyment of food and not the "poor kid" who can't eat anything. After all, in my kitchen, every child gets a cookie!

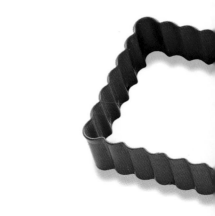

Leslie Hammond

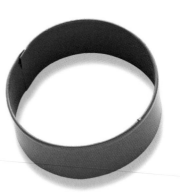

Basics for This Cookbook

I have spent the past ten years consulting, teaching cooking classes, writing articles, and developing recipes. After working with families, and having a large family of my own (some with food restrictions and some without), I decided to choose recipes for this cookbook with three things in mind:

1. **Simplicity**—I want everyone to be able to re-create each recipe. I know that there are a lot of amazing cooks out there, but many moms, dads, and child care providers cannot dedicate their time to create daily masterpieces. Many families have not ventured out from purchasing store-bought cakes to make their own. When their child is diagnosed with food restrictions, many busy parents feel overwhelmed with having to avoid many convenience foods. This book is designed with everyone's cooking level in mind. Plus, all of the recipes are free of gluten/wheat, dairy/casein, tree nuts/peanuts, eggs, soy, fish/shellfish, sulfites, and sesame! There is no need for substitutions.

2. **Convenience**—My goal is for everyone to be able to go to the store and purchase ingredients to create delicious meals for all family members, with cost, ease, and time-efficiency in mind. The recipes' ingredients are chosen by their availability in local stores and the ability to be re-created in a timely manner so you can focus on spending more time with your family, not trying to figure out complicated recipes, blended mixes, and substitutions.

3. **Quality**—All the recipes have been tried and tested with each ingredient variation used. I wanted to deliver the easiest variety of realistic meals, snacks, and treats that the whole family can enjoy, including the family members and friends who do not have food restrictions, without the worries of only finding a few recipes that cater to your allergy needs.

You will find helpful hints, resources, and information in the sidebars throughout the book. Please keep in mind that it is difficult to cater to all food restrictions Although all of these recipes were created without the major allergens (wheat, gluten, dairy, peanuts, tree nuts, egg, soy, shellfish, fish, sulfites, and sesame), I understand that many people have allergies that are not excluded in this book. Please feel free to use substitutions freely to create your own perfect allergy-friendly recipes.

BASIC SUBSTITUTES

I give just the basics in this book. By now you probably know your dos and don'ts in the world of allergies and you're ready to get cooking! I've included a list of a few recommended products that are used in this book and where to find them. Please periodically check the manufacturer's information to make sure they are still allergen-free. I suggest these products for the best outcome with the recipes, but ultimately the choice of products and ingredients that you use is up to you and your physician. Science and availability of products are always changing; for example, I do not use margarine because there are no products currently on the market that are free of dairy, nuts, casein, soy, and/or gluten. Recently, certain medical research suggested that "highly refined oils" do not contain the protein (such as soy or nut) that causes the allergic reactions. Therefore, it becomes a choice between you and your physician whether or not to include margarine in the child's diet. I chose to create this book margarine-free since so many people have to avoid soy proteins.

Let's take a basic look at some main "staple" foods that mainstream "chefs" (aka, moms and dads) use to create everyday foods for their families and find alternatives to them so that we can make our families allergy-safe meals, snacks, and treats! I will also list some my favorite products and where you can get them!

Dairy—Butter, Cheese, and Milk Substitutes
Dairy is an essential ingredient in mainstream cooking and baking. The most common dairy baking ingredient is butter, which adds moistness and richness, assists in leavening, yields good melting qualities, helps to hold the shape of dough, and gives a delicious flavor to your baking and cooking products. Higher fat content dairy, including cream, sour cream, yogurt, and buttermilk, contributes texture, flavor, and color to dough and helps with leavening. Cheese also acts as a thickener and flavor enhancer to many meals and snacks.

Butter
The most common butter substitute is margarine. If you have multiple allergies, margarine is often on your "no" list. For butter- and margarine-free cooking, I use the following:

Non-hydrogenated vegetable shortening—Shortening is a great substitute for butter in many recipes. It helps to make frostings thick and creamy, it gives shape and moisture to baked goods, and it's practically flavorless so it can be used in both sweet and savory baking. Shortenings are often made with soy or can be contaminated with nuts. Contact the manufacturer to ensure safety. I have created all of the recipes using Spectrum Organic Shortening, which can be purchased at most grocery stores and natural food stores.

Expeller-pressed vegetable oil—In many recipes, from cakes to pastas, I rely on oils to add moisture. Try using olive oil in place of butter on your veggies, gluten-free bread, and pasta sauces. I prefer to use organic canola, olive, and safflower oil in my recipes. You have to decide what works best for you. Do note that many vegetable oil blends contain soy. Oils can be purchased at most grocery stores and natural food stores.

Unsweetened organic applesauce—Purchase organic unsweetened applesauce with no added sugar or flavorings. Unsweetened applesauce does a good job replacing butter and fats in baked goods. If you happen to be allergic to apples, replace the amount of unsweetened applesauce with puréed pears, yellow squash, bananas, or prunes. It will change the flavor, but if you need a substitution, give it a try. You can find unsweetened organic applesauce at most grocery stores and natural food stores.

Cheese
Cheese is frequently used to create many main dishes, like macaroni and cheese, pizzas, and cream sauces. Here I replace it with vegetables and allergy-friendly sauces. I have not yet found a cheese product that is free of casein, soy, nuts, or corn. I use my creativity and imagination in this department to thicken and flavor some of my favorite dishes with allergy-free pizzazz. To replace buttermilk, sour cream, cheeses, sauces, and yogurt, I use the following:

Rice milk and tapioca starch—This blend is easy to make, and the ingredients are easily attainable.

Bean purées—These can act as a substitute for many creamy dairy bases.

Vegetables and spices—Get creative with these healthful ingredients to make delicious recipes where you won't even miss the cheese.

Milk
You can select your own alternatives to dairy, nut, and soy milks. I use rice milk. There are many milk alternatives on the market, like hemp milk and gluten-free oat milk. Make sure you contact the manufacturer to check for contamination. Milk alternatives can be purchased at most grocery stores and natural food stores.

Wheat/Gluten—Flour, Grains, Pastas, Bread, Cookies, and Crackers
Wheat flour helps to bind baked goods like cookies and cakes. Gluten is the protein that gives bread the ability to rise properly and hold its shape in cooking. Wheat flour is soft and smooth to the tongue.

Flour
Flour is made from grains generally containing gluten (wheat, rye, barley, cake flour, graham, etc.). Flour is in most everything edible that you buy. It is even lurking in foods that you might never expect it to be in! If you are going wheat/gluten free, make sure to inspect your packaged goods and read the labels on everything! Look for the Certified Gluten-Free logo on your packages. For added safety, contact the manufacturer and ask about the contamination risks of gluten in the product.

I have heard a lot of families express concerns regarding their children's fiber and nutrient intake while eating a celiac or allergen-free diet. I prefer using brown and white rice flours, rice bran, non-gluten-contaminated oats, and flax meal/seeds, all of which provide fiber and important nutrients. All of these items are easily attainable at most grocery markets, reasonably priced, and produce a quality finished product.

There are a variety of flours available, such as sorghum, pea, bean, and other allergy-friendly flours that you can mix together to make a gluten-free baking blend. Many flours are higher in protein and add more nutrients to your baked goods than even wheat flour. They also have a very strong, distinctive flavor, which is great for some recipes, but the strong flavors do not complement some sweeter, more delicately flavored cookies and cakes.

For my family, I prefer using brown and white rice flours. They are easy to digest, and the flavor is very mild and lets my baked goods taste similar to the wheat versions. If you are concerned about nutrients, there are plenty of safe foods that deliver the health benefits that your family needs: vegetables, fruits, lean proteins, and whole grains like gluten-free brown and wild rice. My pediatrician recommends a daily multivitamin for my kids as well. Consult your doctor for the right allergen-free vitamin for your family.

When it comes to things like cakes and cookies, my focus is on something delicious and fun. These treats come after my family has had its nutritious meal. I want to be able to taste the batter, lick the mixing spoon, and savor the flavor of the goodie that I created. I find that rice flour works perfectly for that! White and brown rice flour can be used alone or mixed together with tapioca flour. I find this combination indispensable for baking without gluten, dairy, and eggs.

Grains

Grains are an important part of our diets, and it's still possible to avoid gluten and enjoy some delicious and nutritious grains available at many grocery stores, natural food stores, and online.

Rice—White and brown varieties, wild, mixed, cream of rice, rolled rice flakes, and rice cereals

Heartier grains—Flax (meal and seeds), sorghum, teff, millet, quinoa (flakes and flour), buckwheat (flakes and flour), and certified gluten-free oats (flakes, meal, cereal, and flour)

Pastas

Pasta is a staple food for many families. There are a variety of excellent gluten-free pastas on the market. They come in all different shapes and sizes, from noodle shapes to lasagna. Check with the manufacturer about contamination of other potential allergens.

DeBoles—This company offers spirals, penne, and noodle shapes that make great cold salads and are perfect with sauces. It is available in most stores if requested.

Tinkyada— This company makes all noodle shapes. This is my favorite pasta because it's easy to make and the most wheat-like in taste and texture. It is available in natural food stores and some large grocery stores. Try to get a hold of their lasagna noodles; they are awesome!

Lundberg Family Farms—This company makes many pasta shapes. It is available in most grocery stores and natural food stores.

Glutano—This company offers rice pasta in fun shapes like animals and ready-to-go macaroni and cheese (contains dairy). It is available in most natural food stores and online.

The Quinoa Corporation—This company makes Ancient Harvest Quinoa elbows, shells, and spaghetti from the quinoa grain. It is available in most natural food stores and grocery stores.

Bread

Another staple food, bread plays a huge role in a family's daily diet: toast with breakfast, sandwiches for lunch, and rolls with dinner. Breads, including pizza crust, is one of the most-missed items for people with food allergies. Bread needs the gluten protein to help it rise and get the desired chewy texture that we love and miss. Allergy-free breads, in my opinion, are never quite the same as regular breads, but many companies have come very close and have made some great products. Here are some of my favorites. Make sure to check with the manufacturer about contamination of other possible allergens.

Ener-G Foods, Inc.—This company offers tapioca, white rice, and brown rice breads (perfect for grilled cheese, toast, croutons, and bread crumbs). It is available in natural food stores and online.

Glutino—This company carries english muffins (our favorite) and a variety of bagels, breads, pizza crust, and cornbread. You can go online or purchase them at your natural food store.

Kinnikinnick Foods, Inc.—This company makes gluten-free breads and offers sliced variety breads, rolls, hot dog buns, pizza crusts, and hamburger buns. It is available at most natural food stores and online.

Cookies and Crackers

Kids big and small love cookies and crackers. Fortunately, we live in a time where there are now all kinds of great-tasting snacks available online and at many large grocery stores and natural food stores.

Remember that lots of snacks out there are naturally allergen-free, such as fruits and vegetables! But if you're dealing with a cookie or cracker snack attack, here is a simple list of snack foods available in most stores. Not all items listed here are free of the big eight allergens (wheat, dairy, soy, peanuts, tree nuts, fish, shellfish, and eggs), so be sure to read labels carefully.

Arico Natural Foods Company—This company makes gluten- and dairy-free cassava chips in original, ginger, barbeque, and sea salt flavors.

Back to Nature— This company offers gluten-free, soy-free, and some dairy-free rice thins in many flavors.

Edward + Sons Trading Company, Inc.—This company makes vegan and gluten-free brown rice snaps.

Enjoy Life Foods—This company offers gluten-, dairy-, peanut and tree nut–, soy-, and egg-free granola, trail mix, cookies, snack bars, and awesome chocolate chips and bars for baking.

Health Valley Organic—This company makes gluten-free rice bran crackers.

Lundberg Family Farms—This company carries a great variety of gluten–free, whole-grain rice chips: Honey Dijon, Pico de Gallo, Wasabi, Fiesta Lime, Nacho Cheese, and more. Rice cakes vary from plain to sweet to savory.

Robert's American Gourmet Food—This company makes gluten-free Gourmet Pirate's Booty and Smart Puffs in sweet and savory flavors.

BASIC BAKING PRODUCTS

Here are some of the brands I recommend for products called for throughout the book:

Ancient Harvest quinoa flakes and flour

Celifibr Pastariso bouillon cubes

Cream Hill Estates certified gluten-free oat flour and grains

Enjoy Life semisweet chocolate chips and bars

Holgrain Brown Rice gluten-free bread crumbs

Let's Do...Organic tapioca starch (instead of cornstarch)

Muir Glen tomato ketchup

San-J organic reduced-sodium wheat-free tamari soy sauce—it contains soy; you can replace with salt.

S & S Maple Camp pure organic maple syrup

Sunbutter organic sunflower butter, creamy and crunchy varieties

Find these and more at natural food stores or online at www.allerneeds.com, www.enjoylifefoods.com, or www.allergygrocer.com.

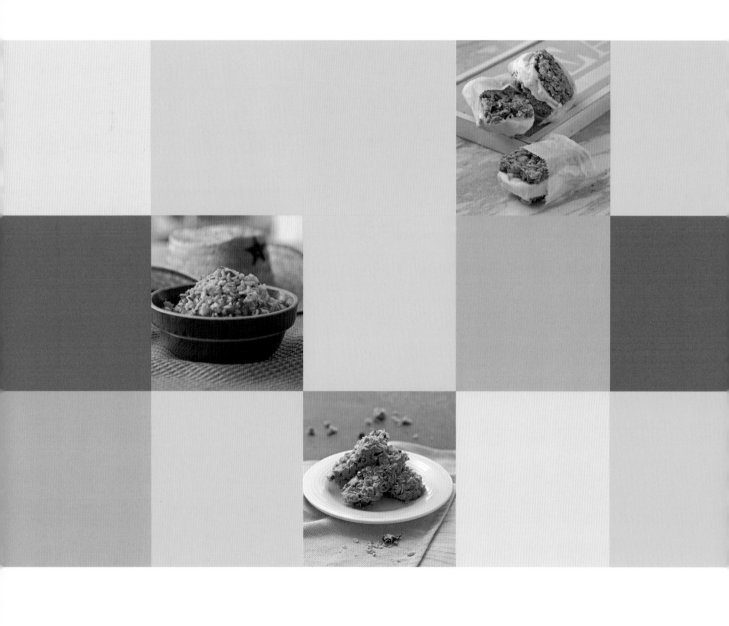

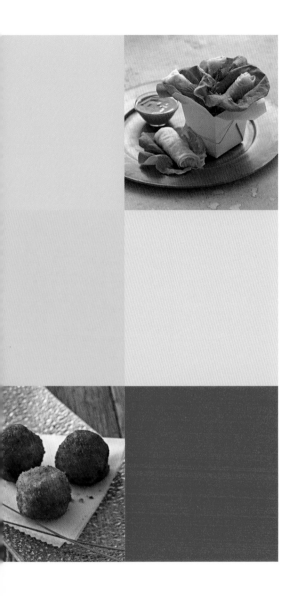

SNACKS and MUNCHIES

Healthy snacks are part of a healthy diet. Children, in particular, need several snacks per day for good nutrition and energy. In this section, you'll find ideas to feed your little ones between meals and munchies for on the go!

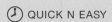 QUICK N EASY

Basic Applesauce

This just in: Apple Eating Great for Your Heart!
Researchers at the University of California-Davis Medical School studied how eating apples and drinking apple juice every day affects heart disease risk. Participants did not change their diets at all with the exception of including apples every day for twelve weeks; in the end, they had reduced their risk of heart disease. Apples contain a variety of antioxidant phytochemicals that decrease LDL ("bad" cholesterol) oxidation. Oxidized LDL cholesterol is more likely to build up in arteries, a process that can cause heart attacks and stroke. So start your child now on a habit of eating apples to ensure a long, healthy life.

1½ pounds (680 g) apples, cored, peeled, and cut into 1-inch (2.5-cm) chunks

½ cup (120 ml) water

1 tablespoon (15 ml) lemon juice

1. In a medium saucepan, add apples, water, and lemon juice. Cook, covered, over medium heat for 10 to 15 minutes or until apples are soft and water is evaporated. Take pan off burner and let cool.

2. Once cool, blend in a food processor or blender until it reaches the consistency you prefer.

3. Cool completely and store in a sealed container for up to one week.

Yield: about 4 cups (serving size ½ cup [120 ml])

18 ALLERGY-PROOF RECIPES FOR KIDS

Blue Applesauce

Basic Applesauce recipe

⅔ cup (100 g) frozen blueberries

¼ cup (50 g) sugar

1. Prepare Basic Applesauce recipe per directions but add berries and sugar at the same time as the apples.

Yield: about 4 cups (serving size ½ cup [120 ml])

A Surprising Muscle Soother
Want to know a great fruit to add to your child's diet if he or she is getting leg cramps or has sore muscles from athletics? The answer is an apple. One medium apple offers 159 milligrams of potassium. Goodbye sore muscles!

Cinnamon Applesauce

Basic Applesauce recipe

2 teaspoons (4.6 g) cinnamon

¼ cup (50 g) sugar

Pinch of salt

1. Prepare Basic Applesauce recipe, adding the cinnamon, sugar, and salt at the same time as the apples.

Yield: about 4 cups (serving size ½ cup [120 ml])

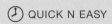

Pink Applesauce

Basic Applesauce recipe

⅔ cup (100 g) frozen strawberries or raspberries

½ cup (100 g) sugar

1. Prepare Basic Applesauce recipe, adding berries and sugar at the same time as the apples.

Yield: about 4 cups (serving size ½ cup [120 ml])

Applesauce Parfait

In my school district, we are not allowed to bring sugary treats to the classrooms. This is a great low-sugar snack that appeals to kids. My experience with kids in classrooms is that they have as much fun with parfaits whether they are made with ice cream or applesauce!

2 cups (500 g) applesauce, homemade or store-bought

½ cup (80 g) frozen or fresh blueberries, strawberries, or peaches

½ cup (60 g) allergy-safe crunchy granola

1. Fill two parfait cups with ¼ cup (60 g) of applesauce each. Layer fruit next, then granola.
2. Repeat the layering, ending with a sprinkle of granola on the top of the parfait.

Yield: 2 parfait cups

A Good Source of Fiber
You've probably heard that an apple a day keeps the doctor away, right? Well, guess what? An apple a day may just help your child maintain a healthy heart for life because the fruit is a great source of soluble fiber. Soluble fiber like pectin, the kind apples contain, actually helps to prevent cholesterol buildup in the lining of blood vessel walls, helping prevent hardening of the arteries and heart disease. So go ahead and eat that apple every day!

Fruit Flowers

This is a quick and healthy snack that kids of all ages like.

  1 large apple or firm pear

  ⅓ cup (87 g) sunflower butter

  1 cup (104 g) any flavor allergy-safe granola or cereal, crushed

1. Wash and core the apple; do not peel. Cut the apple into 8 sections or wedges.
2. Set apple wedges on a plate, peel side down. Spread a thin layer of sunflower butter on both cut sides of each apple wedge. Sprinkle with granola. Serve immediately.

Yield: 1 serving

Breathe Easy with Apples

Here's yet another reason to keep feeding your wee ones those ripe red apples! Researchers in the United Kingdom recently reported that people who eat five or more apples a week have better lung function and lower risk of asthma and other respiratory disease compared to people who rarely eat apples. The ten-year study out of the University of Nottingham examined the relationship between diet and respiratory health in 2,633 people. The researchers suspect that antioxidants in apples lead to these health benefits.

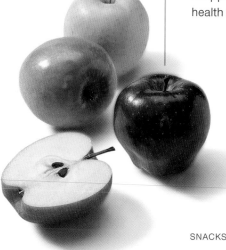

Fuzzy Fruit Ambrosia

Powerful Phytochemicals

As a parent, you know that your children should eat a colorful plate of fruits and vegetables to ensure they receive all the nutrients they need to grow up healthy. But do you know what it is in fruits and veggies that researchers are learning really helps our health? They're phytochemicals! Over 4,000 phytochemicals have been identified and are produced by various plants to help protect them from insects, diseases, and other threats to their health. Those same substances act to protect human health, too. And all we have to do for this health "insurance" is to eat five servings a day!

This festive dish is great for parties. My family serves it as a side dish on Thanksgiving, but we enjoy it as a refreshing fruit salad snack throughout the year because it's a quick way to give a variety of fruits to your kids.

one 15½-ounce (430-g) can pineapple, drained

two 6-ounce (170-g) cans mandarin oranges, drained

1 cup (170 g) sliced fresh strawberries

one 12-ounce (340-g) package shredded coconut

½ cup (120 ml) thick coconut milk (optional)

1. Mix all ingredients together in a large bowl. Cover and refrigerate for at least 2 hours before serving.

Yield: 6 servings

Rainbow Happy Healthy Juice

Proper nutrition is a goal for raising healthy, happy children, but trying to get our kids to eat the recommended daily servings of fruits and vegetables can be a real challenge. I make this refreshing juice with my kids to sneak in both fruits and vegetables to their daily diet. I recommend using organic produce—it tastes better and is better for you. Try creating your own signature mix of fruits and veggies!

3 apples, cored and sectioned

2 oranges, peeled and sectioned

4 large carrots, peeled

½ cup (30 g) chopped fresh parsley

1 pear, cored and sectioned

2 celery stalks

1. Use juicer according to manufacturer's directions.
2. Let children stir the juice and watch the rainbow of colors all combine.

Yield: about 4 cups (serving size ½ cup [120 ml])

Horchata Rice Drink

This Mexican rice milk is a delicious treat. Unlike store-bought versions, when you make your own you can use organic rice, almonds, and berries. Using a small amount of honey adds a touch of sweetness without as much sugar as purchased kinds.

1 cup (200 g) uncooked white rice

3 cups (705 ml) water, boiling

1 teaspoon (5 ml) vanilla extract

½ teaspoon (1.2 g) cinnamon

1 cup (150 g) berries (optional)

Honey to taste

1. Place rice in a food processor. With the metal blade attachment, pulse for about 2 minutes or until rice is powdery. Set aside.
2. Add boiling water to the rice powder. Add vanilla and cinnamon to mixture. Cover and place in the refrigerator for at least 3 hours (or overnight).
3. Transfer rice mixture to a food processor and add berries, if using. Process until smooth. Sweeten with honey to taste.
4. Serve over ice. Keep any unused portion refrigerated and drink within the day.

Yield: about 5 cups (serving size 1 cup [235 ml])

Variation:
Add ½ cup sunflower butter with the berries for added protein.

Nut Allergies

The proportion of children affected by nut allergies has increased dramatically in recent years. Allergic reactions to nuts can range from mild to severe, life-threatening anaphylaxis. Common allergic reactions are as follows:

- A tingling feeling in the lips or mouth
- An itchy nettle rash (urticaria, hives) where the nuts touch you or elsewhere
- Swelling (angioedema) where the nuts touch you or elsewhere
- Swelling in the throat; difficulty in swallowing or breathing
- Asthma symptoms
- Vomiting
- Cramping pains
- Diarrhea
- Faintness and unconsciousness

(Source: www.users. globalnet.co.uk)

Frozen Fruit

Kids won't know that they're eating a healthy snack with these frozen fruit treats—they'll think they're getting dessert before dinner! My children especially like these after a hot day in the park.

- 2 cups (500 g) mashed bananas or applesauce
- 1 cup (200 g) fruit (for example, ½ cup [100 g] each bananas and strawberries or canned peaches and blueberries)
- ¼ cup (60 ml) honey

1. Purée all ingredients in a blender. Freeze mixture in a 9 × 13-inch (23 × 33-cm) casserole dish for 30 minutes. Blend again and pour into popsicle molds or back into the casserole dish. Freeze for 1 to 2 hours.

2. If using a casserole dish, use an ice cream scoop to scoop frozen mixture into balls. Serve with fresh fruit, low-sugar cookies, or allergy-safe granola.

Yield: about 3 cups (serving size 1 cup [235 ml])

Lactose Intolerant? Try Goat Yogurt

Many people who are allergic to cow's milk products or who suffer from lactose intolerance can enjoy yogurt made from goat milk. Yogurt cultures convert lactose into lactic acid, making yogurt easier to digest than milk. According to one legend, yogurt originated when the goat was first domesticated in Mesopotamia about 5000 BCE. Warm goat milk, stored in gourds in the warm climate, naturally soured and formed a curd. According to Dr. Frank Kosikowski, "Someone with sufficient courage tasted this clabbered mass and rendered a favorable verdict. History was observed in the making, and yogurt was on its way." (Source: www.redwoodhill.com/yogurt.htm)

Frozen Yogurt Sandwiches

With these Frozen Yogurt Sandwiches your kids get the best of both worlds—a healthy treat in a fun frozen bar!

⅓ cup (70 g) vegetable shortening

½ cup (100 g) brown sugar

2 tablespoons (30 ml) pure maple syrup

2 cups (200 g) certified gluten-free oats or buckwheat flakes

½ cup (35 g) shredded coconut

1 teaspoon (5 ml) vanilla extract

¼ teaspoon (1.5 g) salt

4 cups (700 g) purchased or homemade frozen Rice Dream ice cream or sorbet, thawed slightly

1. Preheat oven to 375°F (190°C, or gas mark 5). Line two 10 × 15-inch (25 × 37.5-cm) baking pans with parchment paper.

2. In a large saucepan, melt shortening over medium heat, stirring often. Remove from heat and add brown sugar, syrup, certified gluten-free oats, coconut, vanilla, and salt. Mix until well blended. Pour mixture onto one prepared baking pan and press mixture down evenly with a long metal spatula. Bake for about 10 minutes or until browned and bubbling all over. Remove and let cool to room temperature.

3. With a sharp metal spatula, cut into 36 small matching rectangles. Place 18 of the rectangles, smooth side down, side by side in a single layer on the second prepared baking pan to make a firm, large rectangle in half of the pan.

4. Spoon frozen Rice Dream or alternative over the entire cookie surface until it is evenly covered, about 2 inches deep. (If it gets too slushy, refreeze for 10 minutes or until firm.) Place remaining cookies over frozen layer to make sandwiches. Cover and freeze for 4 hours.

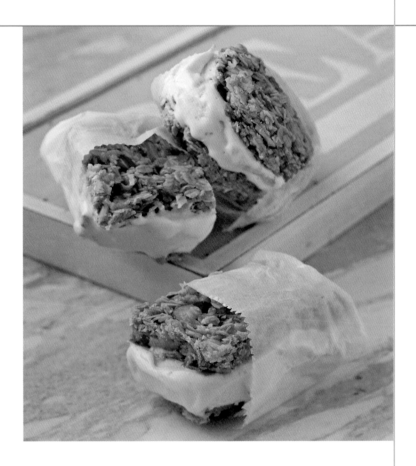

5. Remove sandwiches from the freezer and with a metal spatula cut out each rectangle bar, following the edges of the cookie pattern. Trim sandwich edges evenly if you like. Serve immediately or wrap in parchment and freeze in a resealable plastic bag for up to two weeks.

Yield: 18 sandwiches

The Green Monster Power Smoothie

Natural Gluten-Free Options

Following a gluten-free diet? Don't get discouraged—remember all the whole foods that *don't* contain gluten: fruits, vegetables, rice, corn, nuts, potatoes, red meat, chicken, and dairy products. There really is a world of food out there to feed your wee ones.

Whether your kids are Boston Red Sox fans or not, they'll never guess the secret ingredient in this delicious smoothie. You'll need a good blender for this drink.

2 bananas, sliced

1 cup (235 ml) alternative milk beverage

1½ cups (225 g) seedless grapes, frozen

¼ cup (65 g) sunflower butter

2 green apples, cored and chopped

1 cup (30 g) fresh spinach leaves

Handful of ice cubes

Sugar to taste

1. Place all ingredients in a blender. Purée until smooth. With a spatula, scrape down sides and blend again.
2. Add sugar to taste. Serve immediately.

Yield: about 3 cups (serving size 1 cup [235 ml])

Cool Off Smoothie

This is a great smoothie for a hot day. Allergic to strawberries? Replace with 2 frozen bananas or whatever safe berries you like!

  1½ cups (355 ml) alternative milk substitute or lemonade

  1 cup (300 g) frozen strawberries

  1 tablespoon (13 g) sugar or (15 ml) honey

  1 teaspoon (5 ml) vanilla extract

1. In a blender, combine all ingredients and blend until smooth.

Yield: about 3 cups (serving size 1 cup [235 ml])

Basic Baking Supplies
Remember to read labels on baking supplies like spices, vanilla extract, lemon juice, baking powder, and baking soda. Many of these baking aids are allergen-free, so you have your choice of which brand to pick. Find them at your local grocery stores and natural food stores.

Fruit Basket Smoothie

**At-Home Test for
Gluten Sensitivity**

Perhaps you know your
child responds better to a
gluten-free or wheat-free
diet but no doctor has
ever diagnosed your child
as having celiac disease
or a food allergy. Go to
www.enterolab.com for
more information about
ordering a gluten sensitivity test that you and your
children may take in the
privacy of your home.

Want your kids to eat more fruit? Dip their favorite fruits into this easy,
kid-approved sauce—it also makes a great frosting for cupcakes and
muffins!

> 1 frozen banana, cut into fourths
>
> 1 cup (225 g) frozen mixed berries
>
> 1 cup (235 ml) orange juice
>
> ¼ cup (25 g) flax meal or rice bran
>
> 1 nectarine or mango, sliced

1. In a blender, combine all ingredients and blend until smooth.
   Add more orange juice, if desired, until you reach the desired
   consistency.

Yield: about 3 cups (serving size 1 cup [235 ml])

Whipped Fruit Butter

As far as frostings go, you can't beat fruit for a healthy choice. Try this Whipped Fruit Butter on pancakes and rice crackers, or add some pizzazz to your shortbread cookies, muffins, and cakes. There are no hydrogenated oils or high fructose corn syrups in this delight!

> 1½ cups (225 g) dried fruit pieces (apricots, apples, blueberries, etc.)
>
> ¼ cup (50 g) vegetable shortening
>
> 2 tablespoons (30 ml) honey (optional)

1. Put fruit in the food processor and pulse until fruit is relatively smooth with some chunks. Add the shortening and honey, if using; process for 1 minute or until you reach the desired consistency.
2. Spread on breads or crackers.

Yield: about 2 cups (450 g)

Celiac Disease Resource
Want to find out more information about celiac disease? Interested in meeting with a support group in your area? Visit www.celiac.org, the website of the Celiac Disease Foundation.

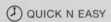

Fruit and Protein Dip

Gluten Intolerance Resource

For more helpful information about managing your child's allergy to gluten, contact the Gluten Intolerance Group of North America by logging on to www.gluten.net.

Though this dip is traditionally eaten with fruit or plain rice crackers, try using it as a filling for a crêpe or a topping for a pancake. It is a healthy alternative to syrup.

½ cup (130 g) sunflower butter or pumpkin seed butter

1 tablespoon (15 ml) honey (optional)

½ firm banana (optional)

⅓ cup (50 g) fresh or frozen berries

Squeezed juice from half a fresh orange

1. Place all ingredients in a food processor and blend until smooth.
2. Refrigerate for 30 minutes and serve with fruit or rice crackers.

Yield: about 2 cups (450 g)

Cinnamon Crunch Snack Mix

My kids call this sweet, low-fat recipe the "ultimate snack."

- 2 tablespoons (30 g) vegetable shortening
- 1 teaspoon (4.2 g) sugar
- 2 teaspoons (10 ml) pure maple syrup or honey
- ½ teaspoon ground cinnamon
- 4½ cups (135 g) puffed rice or corn cereal
- ⅓ cup (50 g) raisins or chopped dried fruit
- ⅓ cup (40 g) pumpkin seeds, sunflower seeds, or shredded coconut

1. Preheat oven to 250°F (120°C, or gas mark ½).

2. In a microwave-safe bowl, melt shortening. Add sugar, syrup or honey, and cinnamon; stir.

3. In a large bowl, mix the cereal, raisins, and seeds or coconut. Pour shortening mixture over cereal mixture and toss until well coated.

4. Pour onto a baking sheet. Bake for about 15 minutes. Stir in the pan, then let sit for 10 minutes and pour into a bowl to serve. Store the leftovers in a resealable plastic bag or a covered container.

Yield: about 5 cups (200 g)

A Honey of a Warning
Do not feed honey to infants under 1 year old—bacteria, which can grow in unsterile products, can cause infant botulism. The same bacteria, however, will usually not affect older children and adults. Curiously, medical researchers in Africa have shown that honey can help clean burns and wounds, reducing the possibility of infection. (Source: *Prevention* magazine's *Nutrition Advisor*)

Crunchy Granola Bars

Low-Sugar Variation:
Omit all sugars, use ⅓ cup (80 ml) sugar-free maple syrup.

Use the crumbs of these bars for a yogurt parfait or chop up the whole batch for a delicious granola cereal. Many families rely on granola bars as a quick snack while running around; these bars are just as delicious as the store-bought ones, but they're made without corn syrups and hydrogenated oils.

½ cup (100 g) vegetable shortening

⅓ cup (70 g) sugar or (78 ml) honey

1 tablespoon (15 ml) pure maple syrup

4 cups (400 g) certified gluten-free oats or buckwheat flakes

½ cup (75 g) raisins (or favorite dried fruit)

⅓ cup (40 g) sunflower seeds or pumpkin seeds

1. Preheat oven to 350°F (180°C, or gas mark 4).
2. Lightly coat an 8-inch (20-cm) square cake pan with cooking spray; set aside.
3. Place the shortening, sugar, and syrup in a large saucepan and cook over low heat, stirring until melted and the mixture is well combined.
4. Remove the pan from heat and stir in the certified gluten-free oats until coated. Add the fruit and seeds; mix well. Pour oat mixture into prepared pan and press down firmly to make a thin, even layer.
5. Bake for 30 minutes. Cool for 30 minutes and then place in the refrigerator. When completely cool, cut with a knife into bars.

Yield: 12 bars

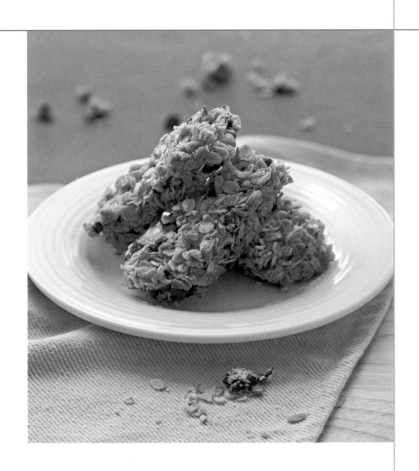

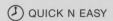

On the Trail Mix

Little hands love digging into this high-fuel snack, best offered on the go.

Low-Sugar Variation:
Use unsweetened
shredded coconut
(and follow the low-
sugar variation for
the Crunchy Granola
Bars recipe).

Crunchy Granola Bars (page 34)

1 cup (70 g) toasted shredded coconut (optional)

1 cup (150 g) chopped dried fruit

1 cup (180 g) raisins

½ cup (15 g) of your favorite rice or corn cereal

½ cup (75 g) pumpkin seeds

1. Crush granola bars into bite-size pieces and crumbs. Mix all ingredients. Keep in a large, sealed plastic container. You may freeze this trail mix for up to 1 month.

Yield: about 9 cups (1 kg)

Basic Trail Mix

This tree nut-, dairy-, and gluten-free snack is the perfect mixture of sweet and salty. I keep a bag in my car for a quick and easy munchie on the go.

> 1 cup (225 g) dry roasted and salted pepitas (pumpkin seeds)
>
> 1 cup (225 g) roasted and salted sunflower seeds
>
> ½ cup (75 g) raisins, dried cranberries, or other dried fruit
>
> ½ cup (85 g) candy-coated chocolates, flaked coconut, or allergy-free chocolate chips (optional)

1. Mix all ingredients in a large resealable plastic bag. Close bag and shake. Ready to go!

Yield: 3 cups (435 g)

Tree Nut Allergy? Try Pumpkin Seeds!

Many people who are allergic to tree nuts can enjoy pumpkin seeds and butters. They're healthy and a good source of omega-6 essential fatty acids (EFAs) and omega-9 fatty acids, compounds that research shows are important for brain development and cardiovascular health. Try using pumpkin seeds and butters for making brownies, smoothies, pesto, or veggie burgers. This opens up a whole variety of possibilities that have the nutty taste you love, but without the allergen-triggering nuts! I suggest Omega Nutrition Pumpkin Seed Butter for a replacement to peanut butter. Order online at www.omeganutrition.com.

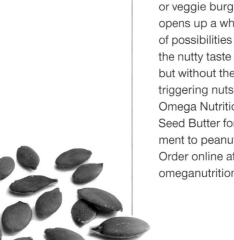

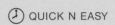

Honey Mustard Snack Mix

**Double-Check
New Products for
Possible Allergens**
Whenever you purchase
a new product from
the store—like chips or
pretzels—I highly recom-
mend calling the cus-
tomer service line and
checking that, indeed, the
offending ingredient isn't
in the product. Ingredients
are subject to change by
the manufacturer. Most
companies list toll-free
consumer numbers some-
where on the packaging,
making it simple to guar-
antee your child won't
be eating something that
could harm him. Inciden-
tally, Ener-G Foods makes
a great gluten-free pretzel.
Go to www.ener-g.com.

Tangy and sweet, this is a lower-fat snack that fulfills your potato chip desires.

2 teaspoons (10 ml) olive oil

2 teaspoons (10 g) Dijon mustard

2 teaspoons (10 ml) honey

4½ cups (135 g) puffed corn or rice cereal

1 cup (150 g) gluten-free pretzels or dried peas (optional)

1. Preheat oven to 250°F (120°C, or gas mark ½).
2. In a large bowl, combine the oil, mustard, and honey. Add the cereal and pretzels or dried peas. Stir to coat.
3. Bake for 15 minutes. Remove and stir. Let the snack mix sit for 10 minutes before serving.

Yield: about 5½ cups (295 g)

Cut Out Croutons

Try cutting these croutons into tiny squares for salads, soups, and snacks or use fun cookie cutters to make giant crunchy treats for toddlers.

4 pieces gluten-free bread

For Savory:

½ cup (120 ml) vegetable or olive oil

2 teaspoons dried seasonings ([0.6 g] parsley or [2.8 g] basil)

Dash salt and pepper

For Sweet:

¼ cup (60 ml) vegetable oil

2 teaspoons (4.6 g) cinnamon

1 tablespoon (15 g) turbinado sugar or (15 ml) honey

1. Preheat oven to 350°F (180°C, or gas mark 4).

2. Toast the bread in a toaster on medium-low heat 3 or 4 times until very dry. Do not let burn. Set aside to cool.

3. In a large bowl, stir together the oil and savory or sweet seasonings.

4. Cut the toast into bite-size squares or desired shapes. Add the toast shapes to the bowl and toss until each piece is seasoned. Add salt and pepper to savory croutons, if desired.

6. Grease a baking sheet and evenly space the croutons on the sheet. Bake for 5 minutes on each side. Remove and let cool on baking sheet for 15 minutes. Serve or store in a covered container for up to 1 week or freeze, if desired.

Yield: about 2 cups (200 g)

Chewy Granola Bars

Beneficial Buckwheat

Buckwheat is a gluten-free grain that has been eaten for hundreds of years in the Far East. China, Japan, Korea, and other Asian countries have long enjoyed noodles made from buckwheat flour. You can also use buckwheat flour in a variety of baked products, including pancakes, breads, muffins, crackers, bagels, cookies, and tortillas. Buckwheat is thought of as a cereal, but it is actually an herb of the buckwheat family, Polygonaceae. It has a distinctive flavor that may not please picky palates, but there are lots of ways to try it, and your kids may find they like it some ways better than others.

Although this recipe calls for chocolate chips, I occasionally use white chocolate chips and dried apricots for a tangy and sweet combination. Both oat and buckwheat flakes are a great source of fiber and have a good amount of protein.

> ½ cup (100 g)vegetable shortening
>
> ¾ cup (150 g) brown sugar
>
> ½ cup (100 g) sugar
>
> 2 tablespoons (10 ml) maple syrup
>
> 4 cups (400 g) certified gluten-free oats or buckwheat flakes
>
> 1 cup (70 g) shredded coconut
>
> ⅓ cup (40 g) pumpkin seeds
>
> 1 cup (175 g) allergy-safe chocolate chips and/or your favorite dried fruit

1. Preheat oven to 325°F (170°C, or gas mark 3). Grease a 9 × 12-inch (22.5 × 30-cm) baking sheet; set aside.

2. In a large saucepan, heat shortening, sugars, and syrup until melted. Stir in remaining ingredients until evenly combined.

3. Spread oat mixture on prepared baking sheet and press into an even layer, making sure the surface is smooth. Bake for 30 minutes. Cool completely and cut into bars.

Yield: 12 bars

Morning Bars

Try blueberry bars with chopped dried apple pieces—an ideal quick morning snack when you and the kids are on the go!

⅔ cup (100 g) raisins or dried fruit pieces (apples, blueberries, or apricots)

½ cup (100 g) vegetable shortening or (120 ml) vegetable oil

½ cup (120 ml) honey

4 cups (400 g) rolled oats or buckwheat

¼ cup (30 g) rolled certified gluten-free oats or buck wheat

1 teaspoon (4.6 g) baking soda

½ cup (60 g) sunflower seeds, pumpkin seeds, or shredded coconut

1. Preheat oven to 325°F (170°C, or gas mark 3).

2. Place ⅔ cup (100 g) of dried fruit pieces in a food processor fitted with a metal blade and process for 30 seconds or until smooth. Add the shortening and process until smooth. Add the honey and blend until smooth. Set aside.

3. In a large bowl, mix together certified gluten-free oats, flour, and baking soda. Stir in the seeds and the remaining 1 cup (150 g) dried fruit pieces. Pour the puréed fruit mixture into the oat mixture and stir until thoroughly combined. If needed, pour half of the mixture back into the processor and pulse several times to combine.

4. Line a 9 × 13-inch (23 × 33-cm) baking pan with nonstick parchment paper. Press the oat mixture firmly and evenly into the pan. Bake for 30 minutes. Let cool for at least 4 hours. Invert onto a cutting board and lift pan to remove. Peel off the parchment paper. With a long, sharp knife, cut into desired granola bar sizes.

Yield: 12 bars

The Need for Seeds
Try substituting pumpkin seeds for nuts in your granola, on top of salads, or when making your own chocolate bars for an added crunch!

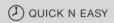

Quick Savory Crackers

Variation:
For an added crunch, add ¼ cup (55 g) roasted sunflower or pumpkin seeds to the dough.

This dough also works nicely for pizza bites and quiches. I feel good about making my family crackers that are free of preservatives and hydrogenated oils.

1 cup (225 g) canned navy or pinto beans, drained

¼ cup (60 ml) vegetable or olive oil

½ cup (60 g) rice flour

¼ cup (28 g) flax meal

¼ cup (30 g) tapioca, corn, or arrowroot starch

⅛ teaspoon (0.75 g) salt

¼ teaspoon (0.65 g) ground cayenne pepper or chili powder

Dash of pepper or dried herbs

1. Preheat oven to 425°F (220°C, or gas mark 7).

2. In a food processor, purée the beans until smooth. Add remaining ingredients and blend until a ball forms and all ingredients are thoroughly combined. Divide dough into 1-inch (2.5-cm) balls. Flatten on a greased baking sheet. Sprinkle with coarse salt. Bake for about 20 minutes.

3. For cracker shapes: Roll dough out to ¼ inch (0.6 cm) on a cutting board. Freeze dough for 10 minutes. Use cookie cutters or let child roll into bread sticks. Make sure all crackers are even in size. Place on a lightly greased baking sheet and bake for 15 minutes. Let crackers cool on a cooling rack.

4. For cut crackers: Roll dough into a log and chill in the refrigerator for 30 minutes. Slice ¼-inch (0.6-cm) slices from chilled log. Bake according to above directions.

5. Store in sealed plastic container or freeze in a resealable plastic freezer bag for 1 month. Unbaked dough may be kept frozen for 1 month.

6. For an added crunch, add ¼ cup (55 g) roasted sunflower or pumpkin seeds to the dough.

Yield: 12 crackers

Herbed Rice Snacks

These are quick and easy to make. My kids like them, and it's the kind of snack that will hold them over until dinner.

1¾ cups (415 ml) water

1 cup (195 g) short-grain brown or white rice

Dash of salt

2 teaspoons (10 ml) honey

2 teaspoons (10 ml) tomato paste

2 teaspoons (3.6 g) dried Italian herbs or (5.2 g) chili powder

1. In a saucepan, combine water, rice, salt, and honey. Cover and cook for about 40 minutes or until rice is very soft. Remove from heat and let stand, covered, for about 10 minutes. Stir in the tomato paste and herbs or chili powder. Transfer to a bowl and let cool for about 20 minutes, stirring occasionally.

2. With damp hands, shape mixture into 2-inch (3.7-cm) balls. Place on a flat surface. Eat warm or enjoy chilled from the refrigerator.

Yield: 3 dozen

Homemade Is Best

It takes more time to cook things that are so easy to buy—but the benefits are rewarding! My children love to participate in the process of preparing most of our snacks and treats. I see that their interest in cooking the foods makes them more inclined to try their new foods. This is especially true if you have a picky eater! Invite your children to scoop out the cookie dough or create their own pizzas with their favorite toppings. I often hear my oldest tell her friends at the park—who are usually eating store-bought crackers—"Taste my cracker. I made it myself!" She is proud of her cooking talents and her gluten-free cracker, too.

Sweet Rice Snacks

These are easy to make, filling, and delicious.

>   1¾ cups (415 ml) water
>
>   1 cup (195 g) short-grain brown or white rice
>
>   2 teaspoons (4.6 g) ground cinnamon
>
>   Dash of salt
>
>   ¼ cup (60 ml) honey or pure maple syrup
>
>   1 cup (150 g) raisins or dried fruit

1. In a saucepan, combine water, rice, cinnamon, salt, and honey. Cover and cook for about 40 minutes or until rice is very soft.

2. Remove from heat and let stand, covered, for about 10 minutes. Stir in the dried fruit. Transfer to a bowl and let cool for about 20 minutes, stirring occasionally.

3. With damp hands, shape mixture into 1½-inch (3.7-cm) balls. Place on a flat surface. Eat warm or enjoy chilled from the refrigerator.

Yield: 3 dozen

Rice Cracker
Personal Pizzas

Kids love creating their own personal pizzas. Just place all the ingredients in front of them and let them go for it! Talk to your kids about healthy choices, portion sizes, and the importance of vegetables as they are topping their pizzas. Give them the gift of nutritional knowledge to help them stay healthy through adulthood.

> 6 rice, corn, or puffed grain crackers
>
> one 14-ounce (395 g) jar of premade pizza or marinara sauce
>
> one 8-ounce (225-g) package of allergy-friendly pepperoni slices
>
> 1 cup (125 g) sliced veggies (pick your favorites)
>
> 1 tablespoon (1.8 g) fresh or dried Italian herbs or basil

1. Preheat oven to 350°F (180°C, or gas mark 4).
2. Place rice crackers on a baking sheet and top with sauce and toppings, including herbs.
3. Bake for 10 minutes or until centers are cooked. Serve immediately.

Yield: 6 pizzas

Cucumber Wheels

If your child has fish and shellfish allergies, sushi is a definite "no." If your family wants to try foods with worldly flair, make this for them instead. This makes a great and easy quick snack.

3 large cucumbers

2 cups (330 g) steamed short-grain white rice, cooled

2 carrots, chopped into small pieces

1 small avocado, gently mashed

½ cup (120 ml) gluten-free tamari

½ cup (120 ml) rice vinegar

2 tablespoons (12 g) sliced scallions

⅛ teaspoon prepared wasabi (optional)

1. Peel the cucumber (or if using a non-waxed cucumber, leave skin on). Cut off each end and then cut in half. With a long, thin knife, hollow out the seeds from the cucumbers. You will have 6 cucumber "logs."

2. In a bowl, mix together the cooled rice, carrots, and avocado. With a small spoon, or with clean hands, fill the hollowed cucumber logs with the rice mixture. Smooth the ends.

3. Using a sharp knife, slice the filled cucumber into 1- or 2-inch (2.5- or 5-cm) wheels. Place on a flat surface or plate.

4. Combine the tamari, vinegar, scallions, and wasabi in a small bowl. Place the bowl in the center of a plate and arrange cucumber wheels around it.

Yield: 6 cucumber wheels

Variation:

If you have super-picky eaters, omit the avocado and carrot and try this recipe with just plain rice and the cucumber. You will be surprised at how even fussy eaters like this.

Hidden Allergens

After a snack or meal, moms everywhere may give the little tykes a bath. But did you know that if your child suffers from allergies, you'll want to read labels on shampoos, bubble baths, and body gels? Many of these products contain wheat/gluten, dairy, and/or nuts in their ingredients and can cause an allergic reaction on the skin of a sensitive child. You can purchase pure glycerin soaps from natural food stores or go to www.wholefoodsmarket.com for a great list of products from beauty to goodies that are allergy-free.

Bean Salad

It is certainly a healthy snack, but this salad also makes a great side dish to any meal.

- one 15½-ounce (430-g) can each black beans, kidney beans, and garbanzo beans
- 1 small red onion, finely chopped
- 1 teaspoon (3 g) chopped garlic
- ¼ cup (15 g) chopped fresh cilantro or basil
- ⅓ cup (80 ml) rice vinegar
- 1 tablespoon (13 g) sugar (optional)
- ¼ cup (60 ml) light olive oil
- 2 teaspoons (5.6 g) celery or poppy seeds
- Salt and pepper to taste
- one 12-ounce (340-g) package frozen fancy green beans, defrosted

1. Drain and rinse all canned beans; set aside.
2. In a large bowl, stir onion, garlic, cilantro, vinegar, sugar, oil, seeds, salt, and pepper until combined. Add canned beans and green beans and stir to mix well. Cover and refrigerate for at least 4 hours before serving.

Yield: 8 servings

Low-sugar variation:
Omit sugar.

Multipurpose Beans
Beans are great! We can eat them cooked, sprouted, popped, and some raw. But you can also use them for alternative flours. Many people use bean flours for a softer texture or added nutrients in their gluten-free cooking. Some popular bean flours are garbanzo, fava, white bean, and even black and green pea flours. However, many people are allergic to some bean flours as well. In that case, turn to flax meal or rice bran in recipes that call for bean flours.

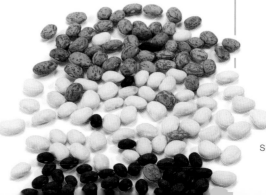

Go Cucumbers!

Celiac Statistics

Celiac disease—once thought rare—has recently been found to be more common, occurring in 1 in 100 Americans, or 3 million people! Diagnosis rates are still low; only 3% of those with celiac disease are diagnosed.

Most parents have to struggle to get their children to eat their vegetables, but my daughter Allison requests this yummy salad often.

  1 teaspoon (6 g) salt

  2 large English hothouse cucumbers, thinly sliced

  ½ cup (100 g) sugar

  1 cup (235 ml) rice vinegar

  ½ cup (30 g) chopped fresh parsley

  1 small red onion, thinly sliced

1. Sprinkle salt over cucumbers on a plate lined with a cotton kitchen towel and set aside for at least 5 minutes.

2. Whisk sugar and vinegar in a large bowl. Add cucumbers, parsley, and onion. Toss together, cover, and refrigerate for 2 hours before serving.

Yield: 2 cups (200 g)

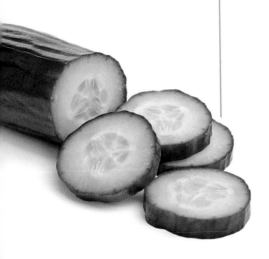

Creamy Veggie Salad

It is almost impossible to purchase deli style potato salad without preservatives and msg. This salad gives you the flavor of the purchased kind but also delivers the goodness of making it from scratch. Potatoes are one of the vegetables that are really important to purchase organic.

1½ cups (355 g) Mock Mayonnaise (see recipe page 163)

2 teaspoons (10 ml) mustard

Salt and pepper to taste

¼ cup (60 g) gluten-free sweet pickle relish

½ sweet white onion, finely chopped

2 celery stalks, finely chopped

5 cups (650 g) combination of your choice carrots, butternut squash, parsnips, zucchini, and broccoli, cooked, cooled, peeled, and cubed

Paprika for sprinkling

1. In a large bowl, combine mock mayonnaise, mustard, salt and pepper, relish, onion, and celery. Gently fold in cubed vegetables. Sprinkle with paprika. Cover and refrigerate for at least 2 hours.

Yield: 5 cups (1.3 kg)

Potato Allergy

Some infants and young children might have an allergy to cooked potatoes that leads to severe allergic disease, according to a study in the September 2002 *Journal of Allergy and Clinical Immunology*. Researchers concluded that allergy to cooked potatoes might be responsible for severe allergic disease in a small number of young children with symptoms of immediate hypersensitivity, atopic dermatitis, or both. This allergy can be controlled by following a potato elimination diet. Source: www.intellihealth.com

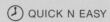
Turkey Rice Salad

Low-sugar variation:
Replace orange juice
concentrate with fresh
squeezed juice.

Want to go vegetarian? Just omit the turkey! Steamed wild rice gives this dish filling fiber.

2 cups (330 g) steamed wild rice blend

1 cup (140 g) diced cooked turkey or chicken

¼ cup (25 g) chopped scallions

½ small red onion, diced

½ cup (90 g) chopped dried apricots or cranberries

¼ cup (30 g) chopped red bell pepper (optional)

¼ cup (30 g) finely chopped celery, including the leaves

¼ cup (60 ml) frozen orange juice concentrate, thawed

¼ cup (60 ml) rice vinegar

3 teaspoons (13 g) sugar (optional)

2 teaspoons (6 g) minced garlic

¼ cup (15 g) chopped fresh parsley

¼ cup (60 ml) canola oil

1 teaspoon (3 g) dried mustard

Salt and pepper to taste

1. In a large bowl, combine cooled rice, turkey, onions, apricots, bell pepper, and celery.

2. In a small bowl, mix remaining ingredients. Pour into large bowl and mix together. Refrigerate until ready to serve.

Yield: 6 cups (1.5 kg)

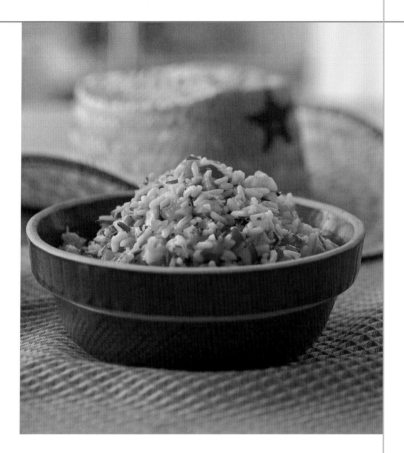

A Surprising Source of Vitamin C

So often we think of fruits as packing the vitamin C punch, but one kind of vegetable offers a wallop of vitamin C: peppers! Sweet green and red bell peppers both provide over 100 milligrams per serving, which is important because vitamin C needs to be replenished every day. And sweet red bell peppers not only are loaded with C but also provide over 2,000 milligrams of vitamin A!

Brown Rice and Apple Salad

Low-sugar variation:
Omit honey.

Swap Sunflower Seeds for Tree Nuts

Sunflower seeds are an acceptable alternative to tree nuts. Check with your allergist to see if this healthy, crunchy peanut alternative will work for your family. Raw, roasted, or as a butter, these little seeds pack a lot of nutrients, including linoleic acid (an essential fatty acid), fiber, protein, vitamin E, B vitamins, and minerals such as magnesium, iron, phosphorus, selenium, calcium, and zinc. Additionally, they are rich in cholesterol-lowering phytosterols. Sunflower oil is one of the more popular oils in the world and can be used as-is or processed into polyunsaturated margarines. In the future, sunflower oil could become a renewable bio-source for hydrogen.

In the summer, try adding 1 cup (160 g) of sliced grapes, strawberries, and/or melon for an added serving of fruit.

2 tablespoons (30 ml) rice vinegar

2 tablespoons (30 ml) olive oil

1 tablespoon (15 ml) honey (optional)

Juice and zest of ½ an orange

2 cups (330 g) cooked, chilled brown rice

1 medium apple, chopped

1 cup (120 g) sliced celery

⅓ cup (50 g) currants

¼ cup (15 g) chopped fresh parsley

¼ cup (60 g) shelled sunflower seeds

1. In a large bowl, mix vinegar, oil, honey, orange juice, and zest.
2. Stir in rice, apple, celery, currants, parsley, and sunflower seeds. Serve.

Yield: 5 servings

Salsa Bean and Rice Salad

Although this is packed with protein, it is a light dish. Many cultures think that the combination of rice and beans is the perfect balance of carbs, proteins, and essential vitamins.

1 cup (260 g) prepared salsa

2 tablespoons (8 g) chopped cilantro

2 tablespoons (30 ml) rice vinegar

2 tablespoons (12 g) chopped scallions

2 cups (330 g) cooked and cooled rice (brown, white, or favorite mix)

1 cup (160 g) corn (frozen, fresh, or canned), rinsed and drained

one 15½-ounce (430-g) can pinto or black beans, drained and rinsed

1 red bell pepper, chopped

1. In a large bowl blend salsa, cilantro, vinegar, and scallions.
2. Stir in rice, corn, beans, and bell pepper. Refrigerate for 30 minutes, and serve.

Yield: 6 to 8 servings

A Connection between Autism and Gluten Sensitivity?

Medical epidemiologists at the Centers for Disease Control and Prevention (CDC) believe that children who suffer from autism spectrum disorders have a genetic predisposition—basically a biological reason—for the disorder but that the "biomarker" or "biological fingerprint" that autistic children possess must be somehow triggered by a pollutant or irritant. Since so many autistic children experience gastrointestinal problems, there are many people who believe that the trigger for some children is gluten or wheat. Although no study has yet proven this to be the case, the CDC is funding a study looking at the prevalence of autism and the possibility of food allergies as a cause.

Macaroni Salad

Fruits and Vegetables in Kids' Diets

According to studies done by the U.S. Department of Agriculture, most kids don't eat a healthy, balanced diet rich in fruits and vegetables. Although dietary guidelines recommend that children over two years of age eat five to nine servings of fruits and vegetables a day, fewer than 15 percent of grammar school children eat five or more servings, and over half of all elementary age children don't eat any fruit at all on a given day. Those children missing out on the servings also miss out on important vitamins and minerals necessary for proper growth. These recipes give you easy, tasty ways to pack produce into your kids' diets (and yours too!).

Macaroni salad has been a favorite of children for generations.

> one 12-ounce (340-g) box elbow macaroni or penne rice noodles
>
> 1 cup (235 g) Mock Mayonnaise (see recipe page 163)
>
> ¼ cup (60 g) sweet pickle relish
>
> 2 stalks celery, diced
>
> 1 small white onion, finely chopped
>
> 1 teaspoon (5 ml) prepared mustard
>
> 1 teaspoon (5 ml) rice vinegar

1. Prepare noodles according to package directions. Cool noodles completely.
2. In a large bowl, combine all ingredients and mix well. Refrigerate until ready to serve.

Yield: 4 cups (600 g)

Noodle Doodle Salad

Macaroni Salad recipe, prepared (page 54)

1 cup (130 g) frozen peas

¼ cup (30 g) chopped bell pepper

one 6-ounce (170-g) can chopped chicken (or freshly cooked, cubed chicken or ham)

1. Mix all ingredients together and serve immediately.

Yield: about 4 cups (600 g)

Variation:
Want a noodle casserole? Forget the boxed version, full of preservatives and high sodium, and make your own! Omit the pickle relish from the Macaroni Salad recipe on page 54. Add the rest of the Noodle Doodle salad ingredients and bake at 350°F (180°C, or gas mark 4) for 30 minutes!

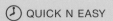 QUICK N EASY

Rice Vinegar Asian Salad

Low-sugar variation:
Omit honey.

Just because they're little doesn't mean they can't appreciate the tastes of the world! My children dig into this Asian-infused snack.

¼ cup (60 ml) rice vinegar

2 tablespoons (30 ml) vegetable oil

1 tablespoon (6 g) minced peeled fresh ginger or 1 teaspoon (1.8 g) dried ginger

2 teaspoons (10 ml) olive oil

2 teaspoons (10 ml) honey

one 16-ounce (455-g) bag prepared coleslaw cabbage

Cayenne or black pepper to taste

¼ cup (25 g) sliced scallions

1 tablespoon (8 g) roasted sunflower seeds

1. In a large bowl, mix together vinegar, vegetable oil, ginger, olive oil, and honey.
2. Stir in cabbage mixture, pepper, and scallions until thoroughly coated. Toss in sunflower seeds and stir.

Yield: about 2 cups (250 g)

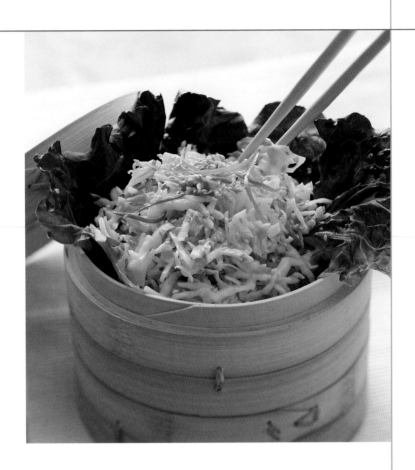

Broccoli Salad

This is one of my favorite salads. It is one easy way to get your kids and husband to eat raw broccoli! Raw broccoli offers many nutritional benefits like vitamin A, C, K, calcium, folic acid, fiber, and iron.

1 head broccoli (about 2 cups or 140 g), rinsed

1 cup (225 g) Mock Mayonnaise (see recipe page 163)

2 tablespoons (30 ml) honey

½ teaspoon (3 g) salt

1 tablespoon (15 ml) rice vinegar

¼ cup (56 g) raw sunflower seeds

½ cup (75 g) raisins or dried cranberries

½ cup (65 g) jicama, chopped into pieces

½ cup (80 g) diced red onion

¼ cup (20 g) bacon bits (optional)

1. Chop the broccoli florets into bite-sized pieces. Chop up some stems if desired. Place in a bowl; fill with very hot water and set aside.
2. Meanwhile, mix the mock mayonnaise, honey, salt, and vinegar in a large bowl.
3. Drain the broccoli and rinse with cold water.
4. Add the broccoli and remaining ingredients to the mock mayonnaise mixture; stir until well combined. Refrigerate for 30 minutes.

Yield: 10 servings

Deli Salad

I serve this deli-style salad on a bed of lettuce with tortilla chips. It's fun for the kids to dip the chips in the salad, and I'm happy because they're getting a helping of low-fat protein. This is a good way to use up leftover chicken or turkey too!

⅓ cup (80 g) Mock Mayonnaise (see recipe page 163)

¼ cup (35 g) finely diced onion

2 tablespoons (30 g) sweet or dill relish

1 tablespoon (15 g) prepared mustard

½ small cucumber, diced

⅓ cup (50 g) diced tomatoes

¼ cup (15 g) fresh chopped parsley

Squeeze of lemon

½ cup (60 g) grated carrot

Salt and pepper to taste

2 cans or freshly cooked and cubed (6 ounces or 170 g) chicken, ham, or turkey, drained

1. In a medium bowl, mix all ingredients together except the meat. Gently stir in meat, coating well.

Yield: 5 servings

Calcium and Dairy Allergies

Many parents worry when their child suffers from a dairy allergy that the child won't receive enough calcium. Calcium, however, is best used by the body with magnesium, and while dairy products are rich in calcium, they offer little magnesium. In order for our bodies to use calcium for bone and tooth health, it must be balanced by magnesium. Foods that give the best ratio of calcium to magnesium usually don't cause allergic reactions! They are green, leafy vegetables like cabbage, brussels sprouts, broccoli, and spinach.

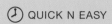

Vegan Salad

Like the Deli Salad, I serve this on a bed of lettuce and let the kids scoop it with tortilla chips. It's a great way to get kids to eat a variety of vegetables.

⅓ cup (80 g) Mock Mayonnaise (see recipe page 163)

¼ cup (35 g) diced red onion

¼ cup (30 g) red bell pepper

¼ cup (30 g) green bell pepper

1 teaspoon (5 g) prepared mustard

½ small cucumber, diced

1 large carrot, diced or grated

⅓ cup (50 g) diced tomatoes

¼ cup (15 g) fresh chopped parsley

Squeeze of lemon

Salt and pepper to taste

1. Combine all ingredients in a medium bowl. Stir gently.

Yield: 1½ cups (225 g)

Thai Rolls

Though more time-consuming to prepare than most recipes in this book, these are a balanced snack of protein, carbs, and vegetables rolled into the perfect size for little hands.

1 tablespoon (15 g) vegetable oil

⅓ cup (50 g) finely chopped onion

1 teaspoon (3 g) minced garlic

1 cup (235 ml) chicken broth or coconut milk

2 tablespoons (16 g) cornstarch or tapioca starch

½ teaspoon (2.5 g) curry paste

2 cups (330 g) Thai rice or wild rice, cooked

¼ cup (30 g) sunflower or pumpkin seeds

8 rice paper wrappers

½ cup (60 g) each carrots and snow peas, cut into thin strips

1. Heat oil in a small saucepan and cook onion and garlic for 3 minutes.

2. In a small bowl whisk broth, cornstarch, and curry paste. Stir into hot onion mixture. Cook and stir until thickened, about 5 minutes. Set ⅔ cup (160 ml) sauce aside. Combine rice, seeds, and remaining onion sauce in a large bowl.

3. Dip each rice paper in warm water and place between paper towels. Let stand for 10 minutes, set aside.

4. Steam veggies for 2 minutes.

5. To assemble each roll, take 1 rice paper and fill with 2 tablespoons of rice mixture. Place some carrot and snow pea strips over rice. Fold rice paper over on each side, rolling up as you would a burrito. Repeat with remaining rice papers and filling.

6. In a steamer, place rolls seam-side down and steam for 5 minutes. Serve with reserved dipping sauce.

Yield: 8 rolls

Helpful Gluten-Free Resource
Are you interested in more information about gluten-related topics, including links to the latest research and articles on gluten intolerance? Check out www.gluten-free.org.

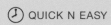

Spring Rolls

Plum Perfect

Plums are a great source of fiber and rich in vitamin A and potassium. So let the little ones dip away at the tangy sauce that's all fruit. Go online to www.honestfoods.com for a variety of gluten-free products like Wok Mei's plum sauce. It's my favorite. As always, check with the manufacturer to make sure that it's free of other potential allergens like shellfish and nuts.

Though spring rolls are traditionally made with rice papers, the wee ones seem to love the large lettuce leaf version as well. Let your kids decide!

4 ounces (115 g) rice noodles, preferably vermicelli

1 cup (75 g) packaged coleslaw salad cabbage mix

⅓ cup (40 g) crushed sunflower seeds

3 tablespoons (12 g) chopped cilantro

1 tablespoon (15 ml) gluten-free tamari

1 tablespoon (15 ml) maple syrup or honey

1 tablespoon (15 ml) olive or vegetable oil

sixteen 8-inch round rice papers or cleaned large lettuce leaves

⅓ cup (80 ml) gluten-free hoisin sauce

¼ cup (65 g) gluten-free plum sauce (or plum jam)

2 teaspoons (10 ml) water

1. Cook rice noodles according to directions. Chop noodles into short pieces.

2. In a large bowl mix together noodles, cabbage, and sunflower seeds.

3. In a small bowl combine cilantro, oyster sauce, tamari, and oil. Pour over noodle mixture and toss.

4. Dip rice papers in warm water one at a time and lay on paper towels. Let stand for 10 minutes.

5. Spoon about 3 tablespoons (45 ml) of noodle mixture onto each rice paper. Tightly roll filled rice paper up from bottom, tucking in opposite sides as you roll. Repeat for each paper.

6. In a small bowl mix hoisin sauce, plum sauce, and water. Serve as dipping sauce.

Yield: 16 rolls

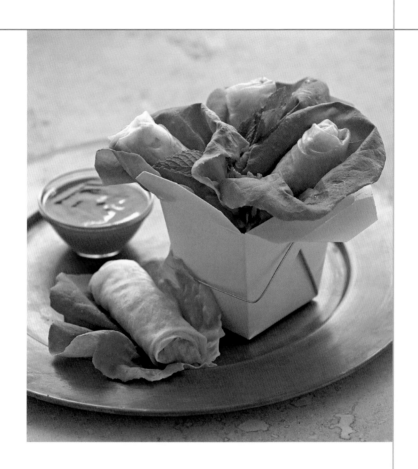

Rice Snowballs

Allergies in the US
According to the National Institute of Allergy and Infectious Diseases, each year more than 50 million Americans suffer from allergic diseases, and allergies are the sixth leading cause of chronic disease in the United States, costing the health care system $18 billion annually.

My only problem with these is that I keep eating them as I go along!

3 tablespoons (45 ml) rice vinegar

1 tablespoon (13 g) sugar (optional)

¼ cup (60 ml) gluten-free tamari

3 cups (500 g) steamed short-grain white rice

1 tablespoon (15 ml) olive oil

3 tablespoons (18 g) sliced scallions

2 zucchini, chopped small

2 carrots, chopped small

2 tablespoons (16 g) toasted flax seeds or crushed pumpkin seeds (optional)

1. In a small skillet, combine vinegar, sugar, and tamari. Bring to a boil until sugar is dissolved; remove from heat. Pour over the steamed rice, stir, and set aside.

2. In the same small skillet, add the oil, scallions, zucchini, and carrots. Cook for 5 minutes or until carrots are tender. Set aside.

3. To form snowballs, scoop about 2 tablespoons (20 g) of rice mixture and form into a ball. Using your thumb, make an indentation and fill with 1 teaspoon (3 g) of vegetable mixture. Cover with rice mixture to re-form ball and gently squeeze with hands; dip into toasted seeds. Cover and refrigerate until ready to serve. You may dip in tamari sauce or enjoy them plain.

Yield: 10 servings

Baked Potato Nachos

The next time you are baking potatoes in the oven, throw in a few extra so you can make this easy meal/snack the next day. Simply double the recipe if you have more people. Organic baked vegetables are a healthier, lower-fat variation to corn chips usually used in nachos.

1 to 2 baked potatoes, cooled and cut into spears
(or zucchini spears or raw jicama spears)

2 tablespoons (12 g) chopped scallions

1 small firm tomato, chopped

Your choice of nacho toppings like olives, jalapeños, and refried beans

1. Arrange the vegetable spears in rows on a greased baking sheet. Broil for about 5 minutes, or until a little crispy.

2. Remove from oven and sprinkle with scallions, chopped tomato, and additional toppings. Return to the broiler for an additional 5 minutes, watching carefully to make sure nothing burns.

3. Remove with a spatula and place spears around a bowl of Sneaky Guacamole (see recipe page 66) or your favorite dipping sauce.

4. If you prefer, you can make your own tortilla chips for nachos by preparing the Bean Tortillas recipe (see page 70) and cutting them into triangles.

Yield: 4 servings

Shredded cheese alternative:
With a small grater, shred a carrot and sprinkle a little over your dish to add a touch of color.

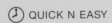

Sneaky Guacamole

Make Food a Learning Opportunity

Want to expose your child to foods of the world? One way to do that is to practice words used by other languages to describe various foods. A French example could include the word *crudités:*

Pronunciation: kr[UE]-dE-tA, krü-di-'tA
Function: noun, plural
Etymology: French, from plural of *crudités* ("raw-ness"), from Latin *cruditas* ("indigestion"), from *crudus*
Definition: pieces of raw vegetables (such as celery or carrot sticks) served as an appetizer, often with a dip. (Source: www.merriam-webster.com)

It can make foods a fun geography and language opportunity!

This is a great way to sneak in an extra vegetable and lower the fat of your basic guacamole. Omit the salsa and this makes a smooth and creamy dip for your little ones. I have even seen picky eaters who do not like chunky guacamole enjoy this.

⅓ cup (90 g) prepared salsa

1 can green beans, drained

1 firm, ripe avocado, sliced

1. In a blender or food processor, add the can of drained green beans and avocado. Blend until smooth. Pour into a dish and stir in salsa.

Yield: about ½ cup (113 g)

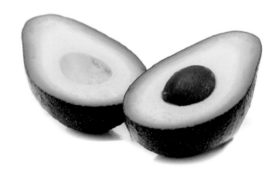

Pizza Bites

Know what's in your pizza bites! You can feel proud to offer your kids a hip, yummy treat made with all-natural ingredients. These may be kept frozen and reheated individually.

  1 recipe Perfect Pie Crust (page 225)

  10-ounce (280-g) jar pizza sauce

  8-ounce (225-g) package allergy-safe pepperoni, chopped small

  1 cup (125 g) of your favorite toppings, chopped small

  2 tablespoons fresh or dried (7.6 g or 2.g) parsley or (5.3 g or 9 g) basil

1. Preheat oven to 350°F (180°C, or gas mark 4).

2. In mini or large muffin tins, place a scoop of dough and press around the sides and the bottom of the tin. Bake for 10 to 15 minutes or until golden and firm. Do not turn off the oven.

3. Remove the dough from the oven and fill each cup with pizza sauce, pepperoni, and your favorite toppings. Sprinkle chopped parsley or basil over tops.

4. Bake for 10 more minutes. Cool almost completely and remove from pan with a spoon. Serve or cool for an additional 10 minutes and then place on a baking sheet and put into the freezer for 30 minutes. Remove frozen pizzas and place into a resealable plastic freezer bag and freeze up to 1 month. To cook from frozen state, place directly into preheated oven at 350°F (180°C, or gas mark 4) on a baking sheet; cook for 20 minutes. Or place in a microwave and cook on high for 3 to 6 minutes.

Yield: 24 pizza bites

Kid-Tested Favorites

When I decided to write this cookbook, I went out to various schools and surveyed children about what their favorite foods were. Overwhelmingly, the kids responded "pizza, nachos, and macaroni and cheese" as among their top favorites. Unfortunately, for a kid with food allergies, all three are toxic to his or her little system. That's why I felt compelled to find ways to feed little mouths their favorite foods—without causing an allergic reaction. Bon appetit!

Hot and Yummy Pockets

This versatile dough is delicious with a variety of fillings. Make up your own healthy creation. Use organic products and lots of veggies!

For Pastry:
1 cup (125 g) oat or sorghum flour

¼ cup (30 g) brown rice flour

¼ cup (28 g) flax meal

¼ cup (25 g) teff flour or rice bran

⅓ cup (80 ml) vegetable oil

½ cup (120 ml) apple juice

Dash of salt and pepper

Olive oil for brushing

For Filling:
1 cup (260 g) spaghetti sauce

1 cup (125 g) finely chopped broccoli, ham, or pepperoni (or combi-nation)

1 tablespoon (4.5 g) fresh or (4.5 g) dried Italian herbs

1. To make the pastry: In a food processor, combine all the pastry singredients and pulse until crumbly. Process until the mixture forms into a ball. Set aside.

2. To make the filling: In a bowl, mix together the spaghetti sauce and broccoli, ham, or pepperoni. Set aside.

3. Pinch off a piece of dough the size of a golf ball. Roll into a flat disk or circle about ⅛ inch (30 mm) thick. You may place dough between two pieces of nonstick parchment paper to make rolling easier. Place a spoonful of filling on one half of the dough circle. With a flat spatula, flip the other half of the dough over the filling to make a half circle with one rounded side and one flat side. Press the tines of a fork into the dough on the rounded side to seal. Repeat with remaining dough and filling. Brush the tops with olive oil and sprinkle tops with herbs. Place about 8 pockets on a baking sheet lightly greased with vegetable oil. Bake for about 25 minutes or until golden all over.

Yield: 24 servings

Mexican Pizza

Store-bought tostadas make this an easy, inexpensive, and totally pleasing snack with plenty of filling fiber.

    6 corn tortillas

    one 15½-ounce (430 g) can refried beans

    1 cup (260 g) mild red enchilada sauce

    ¼ cup (40 g) chopped tomatoes

    ¼ cup (25 g) chopped scallions

1. Preheat oven to 350°F (180°C, or gas mark 4).
2. Bake the corn tortillas for 10 minutes or until firm.
3. Place 3 tortillas on a baking sheet lightly greased with vegetable oil. Divide beans evenly among tortillas. Top with remaining 3 tortillas. Pour enchilada sauce over each tortilla stack. Top with tomatoes and scallions. Bake for 30 minutes. Cut into quarters and serve.

Yield: 3 pizzas

Corn-Free variation:
Replace the corn tortillas with the Bean Tortillas recipe (page 70).

Dairy-Free Cheese
Warning: Be very careful when purchasing dairy-free cheese. Most contain casein and whey or soy potential irritants. Also check to make sure they are gluten-free!

Bean Tortillas

Use this recipe in place of corn tortillas in the Mexican Pizza recipe (page 69) or whenever corn tortillas are called for.

1 cup (225 g) canned navy or pinto beans, drained

¼ cup (60 ml) vegetable or olive oil

½ cup (60 g) rice flour

¼ cup (28 g) flax meal

¼ cup (30 g) tapioca or arrowroot starch

⅛ teaspoon (0.75 g) salt

¼ teaspoon (0.65 g) ground cayenne pepper or chili powder

1. Combine all ingredients in a large bowl. Pinch off a piece of dough the size of a golf ball. With rice-floured hands, roll dough into a ball and flatten into a disk the size of a small corn tortilla.

2. In a frying pan with a dash of vegetable or olive oil, fry tortillas on each side for about 5 minutes over medium-high heat. Remove to a plate lined with paper towels to drain. Repeat with remaining dough.

Yield: 6 tortillas

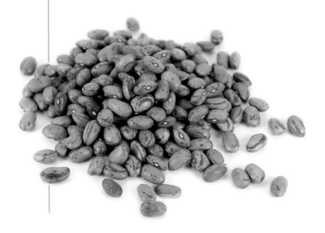

Tortilla Crêpes

These are great for rolled meat, sunflower butter and jelly, and other cold fillings.

  ¼ cup (30 g) tapioca or arrowroot starch

  ½ cup (60 g) rice flour

  ¼ cup (60 ml) canned coconut milk or alternative milk beverage

  1 cup (235 ml) water

  1 tablespoon (15 ml) oil

1. In a bowl, whisk together starch, rice flour, coconut milk, and water. In a small frying pan or crêpe pan, heat a little of the olive oil over medium-high heat. When very hot, pour about ⅔ cup (160 ml) of the batter into the hot pan and swirl around to coat the bottom of the pan evenly. The mixture will bubble up all over, leaving holes covering the entire surface.

3. When the sides of the crêpe start to curl up, lift up an edge with a spatula and check to see if the bottom is browned. Flip crêpe over and brown the other side if desired. Remove to a plate and cover. Repeat with remaining batter. Add a little more oil to the pan when needed.

4. The crêpes will be very crunchy when first cooked, but they soften when they cool. Fill with desired fillings and fold over. If using liquid fillings, wrap the rolled-up crêpe with a paper towel because your crêpe will be full of holes. Store, covered, in the refrigerator.

5. I prefer to eat these crêpes hot. If they need to be reheated, do so in a frying pan to make them crunchy again.

Yield: about 3 crêpes

Mini "Mock" Quiches

These are great because they are a high-protein snack that you can keep frozen and use when needed. I make these in mini muffin tins.

1 recipe Perfect Pie Crust (page 225), unbaked

1 tablespoon (15 ml) olive or vegetable oil

1 cup (150 g) chopped vegetables like mushrooms, squash, and/or broccoli

½ cup (60 g) chopped cooked ham or bacon (optional)

1 cup (235 ml) broth

1 cup navy beans, drained

4 teaspoons (12 g) tapioca starch or cornstarch

Salt and pepper to taste

1. Preheat oven to 350°F (180°C, or gas mark 4).

2. Pinch off a small piece of dough and press it into the bottoms of a mini muffin or regular-sized muffin tin. Set aside.

3. In a large frying pan, heat the oil over medium-high heat and sauté the vegetables and meat, if using, until tender. Fill each tart with the vegetable mixture.

4. In a food processor, pulse together the broth, beans and starch. Season with salt and pepper. Spoon broth mixture over each tart, filling about halfway.

5. Bake for 15 minutes. Remove and let cool to room temperature. Serve warm or place in refrigerator to chill completely. To freeze, place in the refrigerator to completely chill. Place quiches on a baking sheet and put in the freezer for about 30 minutes. When they are able to hold their shape, put all of them in a resealable plastic freezer bag to freeze. They can be frozen for up to 2 months. To reheat, cook in the microwave for 1 minute or until hot.

Yield: 24 quiches

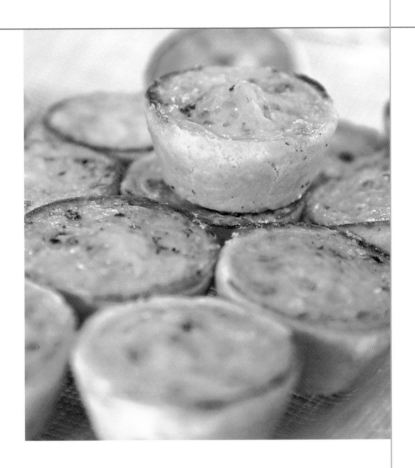

Tempura Veggies

Zucchini Trivia
Explorers brought back the strange vegetable to Europe; in fact, in Italy, it was named *zucchino*, a derivative of our English, "zucchini." No matter what you call it, zucchini offers valuable antioxidants and is rich in potassium, and its mild flavor makes it a kid-friendly addition to all kinds of dishes.

You can batter up almost anything with this, but it especially makes great onion rings.

- 2 cups (250 g) zucchini, onions, sweet potato, or any favorite "safe" vegetable
- 1 cup (235 ml) alternative milk beverage or water
- 1 teaspoon (5 ml) vegetable oil, plus additional for frying
- 1 tablespoon (14 g) flax meal
- ½ cup (60 g) rice flour
- ½ cup (60 g) corn, tapioca, or arrowroot starch
- 1 teaspoon (4.6 g) baking powder
- Pinch of salt

1. Slice vegetables into long, slender spears. If making onion rings, cut into ¼-inch (0.6-cm) slices and separate the rings.
2. In a medium bowl, whisk together the milk alternative, oil, flax meal, flour, starch, baking powder, and salt. Let sit for five to ten minutes.
3. In a large pot, heat 2 inches (5 cm) of oil to 325°F (170°C). Dip the vegetable pieces into the batter. With a slotted metal spoon, lower the battered vegetables into the oil. You can fry 3 to 4 at a time. Remove when golden. Set on a paper towel to drain. Serve immediately.

Yield: about 6 servings

Polenta Snack Cakes

This is a great vegetarian dish ideal for bringing with you when you are going places where you are unsure if the food is allergy-friendly. They taste great hot or cold.

> one 16-ounce (455-g) box 5-minute instant polenta
>
> one 15½-ounce (430-g) can black beans, drained and rinsed
>
> one 15½-ounce (430-g) can corn, drained and rinsed
>
> ½ cup (60 g) each diced red pepper
>
> ½ cup (60 g) each diced red onion
>
> ¼ cup (25 g) chopped scallion
>
> 2 teaspoons (5.2 g) chili powder
>
> 1 small zucchini, shredded

1. Preheat oven to 350°F (180°C, or gas mark 4).
2. Follow package directions for quick-style polenta. Combine cooked polenta with remaining ingredients and pour into a lightly greased large baking dish or muffin pan.
3. Bake for either 1 hour or until firm or 30 minutes for the muffins. Let cool for 30 minutes until firm and either cut into desired size snack cakes or remove from muffin pans. Let cool completely. Cover and keep refrigerated for up to 5 days. They may be eaten cold or reheated.

Yield: 16 cakes

Corn-Free variation:
Combine 1½ cups (120 g) of certified gluten-free steel cut oats and 2 cups (470 ml) of salted water. Bring to a boil in a covered saucepan and then let simmer on low heat for 15 minutes or until oats absorb all the water and are tender. Add additional water if needed. Use oat mixture in place of the polenta and proceed with the recipe as directed.

Corn Substitutes

If you cannot use corn, try the following replacements:

- Corn flour with millet flour
- Cornstarch with tapioca or arrowroot starch
- Cornmeal with flax meal or certified gluten-free steel cut oats or quinoa

"Cheesy" Rice Balls

Cheesy rice balls are a popular appetizer in Italy. I've turned this into a vegan, allergy-safe dish that is equally delicious and sneaks a serving of veggies into your diet. These make a great snack.

    2 cups (330 g) arborio rice, cooked

    2 tablespoons (30 ml) olive oil

    1 cup (132 g) canned pumpkin

    Salt and pepper

    ¼ cup (60 ml) water

    1 tablespoon (8 g) corn, tapioca, or arrowroot starch

    1 teaspoon (5 ml) vegetable oil

    1½ cups (175 g) fine gluten-free bread crumbs

    additional vegetable oil for frying

1. In a large bowl, mix hot cooked rice, olive oil, canned pumpkin, and salt and pepper to taste. Let cool. Form into balls the size of an egg.

2. In a bowl, whisk together the water, starch, and 1 teaspoon (5 ml) vegetable oil; set aside. Pour bread crumbs onto a rimmed plate. Quickly dip each ball in starch mixture (use a slotted spoon if needed) and then roll in bread crumbs until well coated. Set aside.

3. Heat 1 inch (2.5 cm) of oil in a deep frying pan. Fry rice balls until golden brown, turning occasionally. Drain well on paper towels. Serve warm with prepared marinara or allergy-safe dressing as dipping sauce.

4. These do not reheat well and are best eaten the same day you make them.

Yield: 16 rice balls

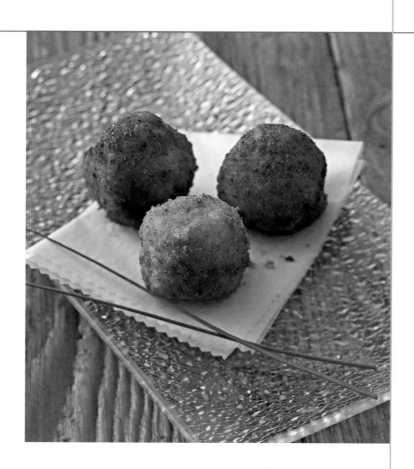

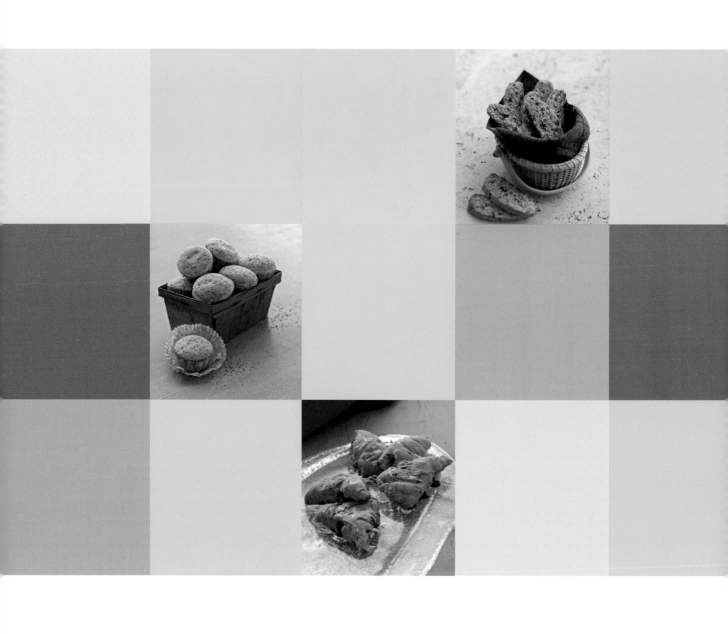

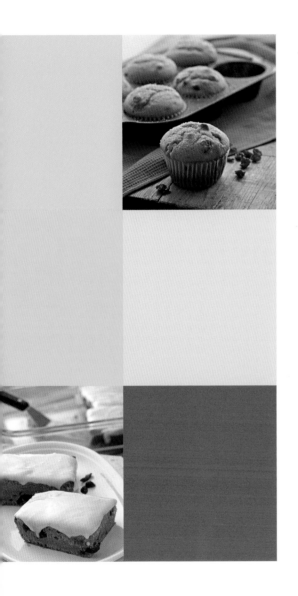

MUFFINS and BREADS

We all love baked goods—whether it's breads, bars, rolls, or muffins! Designed to mimic bakery-style treats, these muffins and bars are easy to make and delicious. Take one and go! I am sure your family will be as pleased as I am with these. Many recipes are a great source of fiber for your family's diet.

Awesome Fluffy Lemon Blueberry Muffins

Berry Wonderful News
In 2001, researchers from Indiana and Ohio State universities found that phytochemicals in red and black raspberries and strawberries inhibit the growth of colon and esophageal cancer cells in rats resulting from exposure to benzopyrene, a carcinogen found in tobacco smoke. While a similar study has not been conducted with humans, there are numerous studies that show that diets rich in fruits and vegetables help reduce the risk of stomach, lung, mouth, colon, and esophageal cancer by as much as 30 to 40 percent. Start fighting cancer early by filling little fists with big, sweet strawberries and luscious raspberries. *Caution:* Some children are very sensitive to berries and should consume them only after the age of two.

Fresh blueberries have high levels of antioxidants and are a good source of fiber, vitamins A and C, folate, and potassium.

> 1½ cups (355 ml) lemonade
>
> 1 cup (200 g) sugar
>
> ¼ cup (60 ml) vegetable oil
>
> 1 teaspoon (5 ml) vanilla extract
>
> 3 cups (375 g) white rice flour
>
> 1 tablespoon (13.8 g) baking powder
>
> ½ teaspoon (3 g) salt
>
> 1½ cups (218 g) fresh or frozen blueberries

1. Preheat oven to 350°F (180°C, or gas mark 4).
2. In a mixer, combine the first seven ingredients (through salt) and mix until smooth. Stir in the blueberries.
3. Lightly grease a muffin tin or line with paper liners. Fill each cup halfway with batter. Bake for 20 minutes, or until firm. Remove and let cool on a rack. Serve at room temperature or refrigerate.
4. For blueberry scones, add an additional 1 cup (125 g) of rice flour to batter. Drop large mounds of dough onto a lightly greased baking sheet and sprinkle with coarse sugar. Bake in a 375°F (190°C, or gas mark 5) oven for about 15 minutes.

Yield: 2 dozen

Simply Delicious Banana Bread

4 medium bananas

½ cup (120 ml) vegetable oil

1 cup (200 g) sugar

2 cups (250 g) white or brown rice flour

½ cup (56 g) flax meal

1½ teaspoons (6.9 g) baking powder

½ teaspoon (2.3 g) baking soda

½ teaspoon (1.2 g) ground cinnamon

Dash of nutmeg

1 teaspoon (5 ml) vanilla extract

½ teaspoon (3 g) salt

1. Preheat oven to 350°F (180°C, or gas mark 4).

2. In a food processor, purée the bananas, oil, and sugar. Add remaining ingredients and pulse until smooth.

3. Lightly grease a 9 × 5 × 3-inch (23 × 12.5 × 7.5-cm) loaf pan with vegetable oil. Pour batter into pan and bake for 60 minutes or until firm in the center.

4. Let cool slightly and then loosen the edges and invert onto a flat surface. Turn loaf flat side down and cool completely. Slice and serve.

Yield: 1 loaf

Skin Reactions to Food Allergies

So often people think that the reaction to food allergies is gastrointestinal or involves respiratory problems. Many food allergies, however, manifest themselves through dermatitis and other eczemas. According to the National Institute of Allergy and Infectious Diseases, health care provider visits for contact dermatitis and eczemas are 7 million per year and seem to be increasing in prevalence.

Lemon Poppy Seed Muffins

Variation:
Omitting the poppy seeds turns these into delicious cupcakes—simply top with your choice of frosting and berries. Or add 1 cup of fresh or frozen berries to the batter and bake as directed.

You can change this muffin to a lemon berry delight simply by omitting the poppy seeds and adding 1 cup (145 g) of fresh or frozen berries. The lemon syrup adds a fabulous touch.

For Muffins:

1½ cups (355 ml) lemonade (or 1 cup [235 ml] water and 1/2 cup [120 ml] lemonade concentrate)

1 cup (200 g) sugar

¼ cup (60 ml) vegetable oil

1 teaspoon (5 ml) vanilla extract

3 cups (375 g) white rice flour

1 tablespoon (13.8 g) baking powder

½ teaspoon (3 g) salt

Grated rind of 1 lemon

¼ cup (30 g) poppy seeds, plus more for sprinkling (optional)

For Lemon Syrup:

¼ cup (25 g) powdered sugar (contains corn starch, use corn-free recipe on page 103)

3 tablespoons (45 ml) lemon juice

1. Preheat oven to 350°F (180°C, or gas mark 4).

2. To make the muffins: In a mixer, combine the first seven ingredients (through salt) and mix until smooth. Add in the lemon zest and poppy seeds and stir until well incorporated.

3. Spoon into desired baking dishes and sprinkle with additional poppy seeds, if desired. Bake until firm: **Mini muffins:** 10 minutes; **Regular muffins:** 15 minutes; **8-inch (20-cm) cake pan or Bundt pan:** 45 minutes.

4. To make the lemon syrup: Add powdered sugar and lemon juice to a small saucepan. Bring mixture to a boil over low heat and then remove from heat. As soon as the muffins come out of the oven, spoon or brush the lemon syrup over the tops. For a Bundt cake, when cake has cooled, invert cake out of pan and pour syrup over top.

Yield: 12 muffins

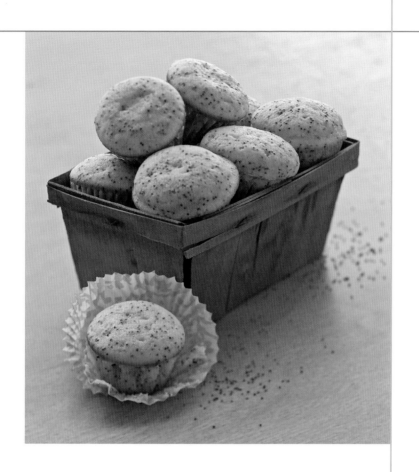

Millet and Currant Muffins

Hope for Soy Allergies
Soybeans are used in everything from ink to baby formula, but many people are allergic to the bean (specifically, a protein within the bean's makeup). Scientists, however, have found out how to "shut off" the gene that makes the allergenic protein in the crop's seed. According to *Agricultural Research* (September 2002), plant physiologists have knocked out this dominant human allergen using biotechnology. Soybeans, along with eggs, milk, peanuts and tree nuts, wheat, fish, and shellfish are considered one of the "big eight" food allergens.

1 cup (235 ml) honey

1 cup (235 ml) plain yogurt or alternative milk beverage

¾ cup (125 g) brown rice flour

¼ cup (28 g) ground flaxseeds

1 cup (140 g) yellow cornmeal

1 tablespoon (13.8 g) baking powder

½ teaspoon (3 g) salt

1 teaspoon (2.3 g) cinnamon

1 cup (150 g) currants

1. Preheat oven to 375°F (190°C, or gas mark 5).

2. In a mixer, blend together the honey, flax meal, and milk alternative. Add in the flour, ground sunflower seeds, millet, baking powder, salt, and cinnamon. Mix until smooth. Stir in currants by hand.

3. Grease a muffin tin or line with paper cups. Divide mixture evenly among muffin cups. Bake for 15 minutes or until firm.

Yield: 12 muffins

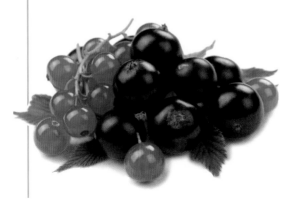

Sunny Cinnamon Bread

1 cup (200 g) sugar

3 cups (375 g) white rice flour

½ teaspoon (2.3 g) baking soda

1 tablespoon (14 g) baking powder

½ teaspoon (3 g) salt

¼ cup (60 ml) vegetable oil

1⅔ cups (400 ml) alternative milk beverage

2 teaspoons (4.6 g) cinnamon, divided

¾ cup (170 g) raw sunflower seeds, ground

¼ cup (50 g) superfine sugar

1. Preheat oven to 350°F (180°C, or gas mark 4).

2. In a mixer, combine the sugar, rice flour, baking soda, baking powder, salt, oil, milk alternative, and 1 teaspoon cinnamon. Mix until smooth. Add in the ground sunflower seeds. Spoon into a greased 9-inch (23-cm) baking pan.

3. Mix the ¼ cup (50 g) superfine sugar and remaining 1 teaspoon cinnamon. Sprinkle over the top of the cake.

4. Bake for 40 minutes or until firm. Cut into squares.

Yield: 12 pieces

Blueberry Coffee Cake

Coconut Controversy

Whether coconut should be considered a tree nut is a matter of some debate. The FDA mandates that coconut be considered a tree nut for labeling purposes; however, as the Food Allergy and Anaphylaxis Network notes, coconut allergies are exceedingly rare, with fewer than 10 reported cases. A study in the *Annals of Allergy, Asthma, and Immunology* indicated cross-reactivity between coconuts, walnuts, and hazelnuts in one patient. Talk to your allergist so he or she can advise you on the suitability of coconut in your diet.

2⅓ cup (290 g) rice flour, divided

¾ cup (170 g) vegetable shortening, divided

½ cup (115 g) brown sugar

1 cup (70 g) shredded coconut (optional)

1 teaspoon (2.3 g) ground cinnamon

2½ teaspoons (11.5 g) baking powder

½ teaspoon (3 g) salt

¾ cup (150 g) sugar

1 cup (235 ml) alternative milk beverage

2 cups (290 g) fresh or frozen blueberries

1. Preheat oven to 375°F (190°C, or gas mark 5).

2. In a food processor, combine ⅓ cup (40 g) flour, ¼ cup (56 g) shortening, brown sugar, coconut (if using), and cinnamon. Pulse until you have a crumbly mixture for topping. Set aside.

3. Grease and flour a 9 × 13 × 2-inch (23 × 33 × 5-cm) baking pan, two 12-cup muffin tins, or a 9-inch (23-cm) springform pan.

4. In a mixer, add remaining 2 cups (250 g) of flour and remaining ingredients except for blueberries. Mix until smooth. Fold in blueberries.

5. Pour batter into prepared cake pan or muffin tins. Sprinkle topping over batter. Bake for 40 minutes for cake or 15 minutes for muffins. Cool slightly. Serve warm or at room temperature.

Yield: 12 slices

Nutty Banana Chip Muffins

I omit the chocolate chips and the sugar and make this muffin at least once a week! The sunflower butter delivers an excellent amount of protein for a little muffin.

4 bananas

½ cup (100 g) sugar

½ cup (120 g) sunflower butter

½ cup (120 ml) alternative milk beverage

2 cups (250 g) white or brown rice flour

2 teaspoons (9.2 g) baking powder

1 teaspoon (4.6 g) baking soda

1 cup (90 g) allergy-friendly chocolate chips (optional)

1. Preheat oven to 350°F (180°C, or gas mark 4).
2. In a food processor, add bananas, sugar, and sunflower butter. Blend until smooth.
3. Add milk alternative, flour, baking powder, and baking soda and blend until combined. Add chocolate chips and pulse twice.
4. Pour batter in your choice of tins and bake:

   Mini muffins: 8 minutes

   Regular muffins: 11 to15 minutes

   Mini loaves: 10 minutes

   Bread loaves: 45 minutes

Yield: 24 mini muffins

Very Berry Scones

¼ cup (50 g) superfine sugar

½ cup (60 g) unsweetened applesauce

¼ cup (50 g) vegetable shortening

2 teaspoons (9.2 g) baking powder

Dash of salt

1 teaspoon (5 ml) vanilla extract

1½ cups (185 g) white rice flour

½ cup (65 g) corn, tapioca, or arrowroot starch

½ cup (120 ml) alternative milk beverage

1 teaspoon (1.7 g) lemon zest (optional)

1 cup (145 g) fresh blueberries, raspberries, blackberries, or sliced strawberries (or a combination)

Raw sugar, for sprinkling

1. Preheat oven to 375°F (190°C, or gas mark 5).

2. In a mixer combine the sugar and the next 9 ingredients (through zest) and mix on low. Increase speed to medium for 1 minute. Stir in the blueberries by hand.

3. Use a medium ice cream/cookie scoop and drop dough on a greased cookie sheet or divide dough into two pieces and form into balls. Place one dough ball on a flat surface. Use a rolling pin to flatten dough into a thick, round disk. Cut dough into 8 mini triangles (like pie or pizza slices). Repeat with remaining dough ball.

4. Grease a baking sheet or line with nonstick parchment paper or aluminum foil. Place about 6 to 8 scones on prepared baking sheet. Sprinkle with raw sugar or brush with additional rice milk.

5. Bake for 25 to 30 minutes or until bottoms are golden and centers feel firm to the touch. Let sit on baking sheet for 1 minute. Remove to a flat surface to cool. These are best served warm.

Yield: 6 to 8 scones

Bran and Raisin Muffins

½ cup (100 g) canned crushed pineapple, undrained

¼ cup (85 g) molasses

1½ cups (150 g) rice or oat bran

1 teaspoon (5 ml) vanilla extract

½ cup (75 g) raisins

½ cup (120 ml) vegetable oil

½ teaspoon (1.2 g) cinnamon

1 cup (125 g) rice flour

1 teaspoon (4.6 g) baking powder

½ teaspoon (2.3 g) baking soda

½ teaspoon (3 g) salt

1 carrot or apple, shredded (optional)

1. Preheat oven to 400°F (200°C, or gas mark 6).

2. Strain the juice from a can of crushed pineapple and reserve ½ cup (120 ml). Combine the juice, pineapple, molasses, bran, vanilla, raisins, and the oil. Let sit for 10 minutes.

3. Combine the cinnamon, flour, baking powder, baking soda, and salt in a large bowl. Add pineapple mixture and stir to combine. Add the carrot, if using, and stir.

4. Line a muffin tin with paper liners. Fill three-quarters full with batter and bake for 35 minutes or until firm.

Yield: 20 muffins

Raisins: Nature's Candy
It is believed that humans discovered raisins when they happened upon grapes drying on a vine. Whether you like yours golden or dark, sweet and chewy raisins make an excellent healthy alternative to candy for the little ones any day! Just remember: Anything sticky and sweet requires a thorough tooth-brushing after eating.

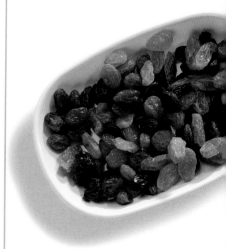

Autumn Muffins

Sneak a veggie into their sweet muffin with this recipe. With or without frosting, these muffins are so wonderful! I recommend the Orange Vanilla frosting on page 230.

½ cup (100 g) sugar (optional)

⅔ cup (150 g) brown sugar

¾ (175 ml) cup oil

2 cups (420 g) canned pumpkin or mashed sweet potato

3 cups (375 g) white or brown rice flour

2 teaspoons (9.2 g) baking soda

2 teaspoons (9.2 g) baking powder

½ teaspoon (3 g) salt

1 teaspoon (1.8 g) ground ginger

1 teaspoon (2.3 g) ground cinnamon

¾ cup (120 g) dried cranberries

¼ cup (56 g) pumpkin seeds

1. Preheat oven to 350°F (180°C, or gas mark 4).
2. With a mixer, combine sugars and oil in a large bowl. Add the pumpkin or sweet potato and mix until smooth. Stir in flour, baking soda, baking powder, salt, ginger, and cinnamon. Mix until smooth. Remove bowl from mixer and stir in cranberries and pumpkin seeds.
3. Pour batter into paper-lined muffin tins and bake for 20 to 25 minutes or until firm.
4. Cool on a cooling rack and frost if desired. Store in a covered container in the refrigerator.

Yield: 24 muffins

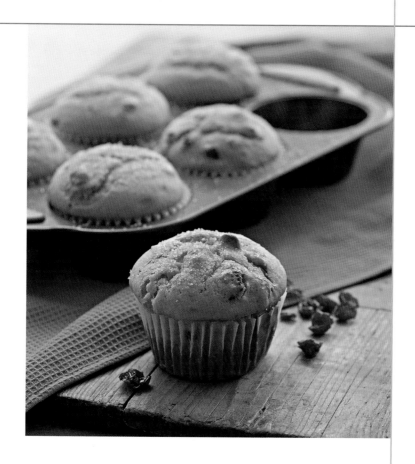

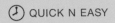

Berry Mini Muffins

Cherry Good!

One cup (110 g) of cherries—besides being incredibly tasty and sweet and a kid favorite—provides 3 grams of fiber, 12 percent of the recommended daily amount. Interestingly, cherries also are packed with protein for a little fruit: one cup offers 2 grams of protein. Try to purchase organic when possible. If buying dried, look for sulfite-free varieties.

¼ cup (32 g) corn, tapioca, or arrowroot starch

½ cup (60 g) white rice flour

½ cup (90 g) cream of rice cereal

½ cup (120 ml) alternative milk beverage

2 teaspoons (9.2 g) baking powder

½ teaspoon (3 g) salt

¼ cup (60 ml) vegetable oil

¼ cup (50 g) sugar

1 cup (145 g) fresh or frozen berries, blueberries, crushed strawberries, pitted cherries, blackberries, or raspberries

1. Preheat oven to 375°F (190°C, or gas mark 5).

2. In a large bowl, combine the starch, flour, cereal, milk alternative, baking powder, salt, oil, and sugar. Gently stir until you have a smooth batter. Let sit for 1 minute. Stir in the berries.

3. Lightly grease or line a mini muffin tin with paper liners. Fill muffin cups three-quarters full with the batter. Bake for 15 minutes. Cool for 10 minutes and turn muffins out on a wire rack to cool completely. Run a butter knife around rim to help release muffins out of tin, if needed.

Yield: 24 mini muffins

Tropical Muffins

These are made with no added sugar and are a good source of potassium.

    3 to 4 ripe bananas

    2 cups (250 g) rice flour

    2 teaspoons (9.2 g) baking powder

    1 teaspoon (4.6 g) baking soda

    1 cup (250 g) crushed pineapple, with juice

    1¼ cups (90 g) shredded coconut, divided (optional)

    2 teaspoons (3.4 g) orange zest

    ½ teaspoon (3 g) salt

    ⅓ cup (80 ml) orange juice

    1 banana, thinly sliced

1. Preheat oven to 350°F (180°C, or gas mark 4).

2. In a food processor, add the mashed bananas, flour, baking powder, baking soda, pineapple and juice, 1 cup (70 g) coconut, orange zest, and salt. Process until smooth.

3. Pour batter into a paper-lined muffin pan and sprinkle tops with ⅛ cup (10 g) coconut. Bake for 25 minutes. Remove to a cooling rack. Arrange banana slices and remaining ⅛ cup (10 g) shredded coconut over the top for decorations. Serve. If you are storing muffins, do not apply banana slices until you are ready to serve.

Yield: 16 muffins

Mini Scones
with Maple Drizzles

You have your choice of pumpkin or apple scones with this recipe. Both pumpkin and applesauce add fiber, vitamins, and antioxidants. They taste even better the next day!

For Scones:

½ cup (125 g) vegetable shortening

¼ cup (55 g) brown sugar

3 cups (375 g) rice flour, divided

¼ cup (60 ml) maple syrup (optional)

1 tablespoon (13.8 g) baking powder

1 teaspoon (2.3 g) cinnamon

Dash of nutmeg

½ teaspoon (3 g) salt

1 cup (250 g) canned pumpkin or applesauce

1 cup (150 g) chopped apples, dried cranberries or raisins

Sugar for sprinkling (optional)

For Maple Drizzle:

½ cup (60 g) powdered sugar (contains corn starch, use corn-free recipe on page 103)

Pure maple syrup, enough to reach desired consistency

1. Preheat oven to 375°F (190°C, or gas mark 5).
2. To make the scones: In a food processor, add the shortening, brown sugar, and 1 cup (125 g) of flour. Process until combined. Add remaining 2 cups (250 g) flour and next 6 ingredients (through pumpkin or applesauce) and blend until smooth. Pour dough into a large bowl and stir in dried fruit.
3. On a floured surface, scoop out a handful-size portion of dough and form into a disk. Using a knife, cut into pizza-like triangles of equal size. Place triangles on a greased baking sheet. Sprinkle with sugar. Bake for 20 minutes or until lightly golden on the bottom. Remove to a cooling rack.

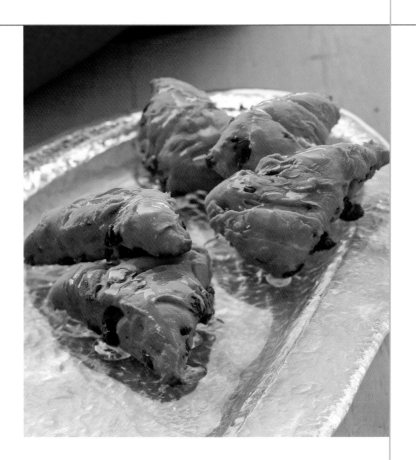

4. To make the maple drizzle: Combine powdered sugar and enough maple syrup to reach desired consistency. Drizzle over scones and serve.

Yield: 24 scones

Banana Crunch Muffins

2 tablespoons (30 ml) vegetable oil

2 tablespoons (30 g) brown sugar

2 tablespoons (30 ml) honey

2 tablespoons (14 g) flax meal

2 tablespoons (30 ml) water

1 ripe banana, sliced

1 teaspoon (5 ml) vanilla extract

½ cup (60 g) white or brown rice flour or sorghum flour

2 tablespoons (15 g) tapioca flour

1 teaspoon (2.3 g) ground cinnamon

1⅓ cups (140 g) allergy-safe granola or cereal

1 cup (150 g) allergy-safe trail mix, any flavor

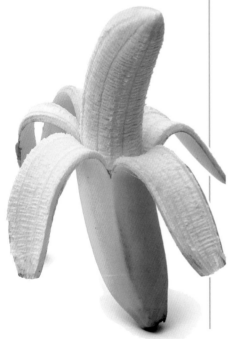

1. Preheat oven to 350°F (180°C, or gas mark 4).

2. In a mixer, cream together the first 7 ingredients (through vanilla). Mix in flours and cinnamon until smooth. If desired, place granola in a plastic bag and gently crush with a rolling pin into bite-sized pieces. Stir granola and trail mix into batter. Spoon batter into a greased or paper-lined cake or mini muffin pan and bake as follows:

   Mini muffins: 30 minutes

   Regular muffins: 20 minutes

3. Cool and cut into small bars or remove from muffin pan.

Yield: 24 bars or muffins

Carrot Crunch Bars

Make this in a jiffy by purchasing pre-shredded carrots.

For Bars:

¾ cup (95 g) brown rice flour

¼ cup (28 g) flax meal

1 teaspoon (2.3 g) cinnamon

¾ cup (170 g) brown sugar

½ cup (120 ml) sunflower oil

½ teaspoon (2.3 g) baking powder

½ teaspoon (2.3 g) baking soda

½ cup (60 g) finely grated carrots

⅓ cup (23 g) shredded coconut

¼ cup raw (56 g) sunflower seeds

For Topping:

½ cup (35 g) shredded coconut (optional)

½ cup (115 g) brown sugar

½ cup (112 g) vegetable shortening

1 teaspoon (2.3 g) cinnamon

2 tablespoons (28 g) raw sunflower seeds

1. Preheat oven to 350°F (180°C, or gas mark 4).

2. To make the bars: Mix flour, flax, cinnamon, brown sugar, oil, baking powder, and baking soda in a bowl. Fold in carrots, coconut, and sunflower seeds. Pour into an 8-inch (20-cm) square greased baking pan.

3. To make the topping: In a food processor, pulse together the topping ingredients until crumbly. Sprinkle over the top of the cake. Bake for 20 minutes. Let cool in the pan and cut into rectangles.

Yield: 12 bars

Frosted Pumpkin Bars

Pumpkin is delicious and nutritious; don't limit this recipe to only holiday use!

For Bars:

1 cup (225 g) canned pumpkin

½ cup (120 ml) vegetable oil

¾ cup (170 g) brown or raw sugar

1 cup (125 g) rice flour

1 teaspoon (4.6 g) baking powder

1 teaspoon (2.3 g) cinnamon

¼ teaspoon (1.5 g) salt

½ cup (75 g) raisins or dried cranberries (optional)

For Frosting:

¼ cup (50 g) vegetable shortening

1½ cup (150 g) powdered sugar (contains corn-starch, use corn-free recipe on page 103)

1 teaspoon (5 ml) vanilla

1 tablespoon (15 ml) alternative milk beverage

1. Preheat oven to 350°F (180°C, or gas mark 4).

2. To make the bars: Mix together the pumpkin, oil, and sugar. Add remaining bar ingredients and mix until batter is smooth. Pour batter into a greased 9-inch (22.5-cm) square cake pan. Bake for 20 to 25 minutes or until firm. Cool completely.

3. To make the frosting: Mix together the shortening, powdered sugar, vanilla, and milk alternative until smooth. Frost top of cooled cake and cut into bars.

Yield: 18 bars

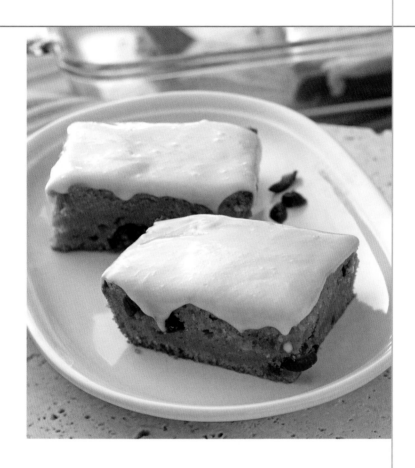

Sponge Cake Slices

Fantastic Flax

One tablespoon of ground flaxseeds and three tablespoons of water may serve as a replacement for one egg in baking by binding the other ingredients together. Flaxseeds come in two basic varieties, brown and yellow or golden, with most types having similar nutritional values. One tablespoon (7 g) of ground flaxseed (about 1 serving) supplies about 37 calories, 3 grams of fat, 2 grams of fiber, and 1.2 grams of protein. Flaxseeds contain high levels of lignans and healthful omega-3 fatty acids. Lignans may benefit the heart and possess anti-cancer properties. Whole flaxseeds keep indefinitely, but you need to grind them to access their health benefits. Grind only what you need and use immediately or refrigerate ground flax meal and store in sealed containers to keep from becoming rancid.

1 cup (125 g) brown rice flour

¾ cup (84 g) flax meal

1 tablespoon (13.8 g) baking powder

¾ cup (75 g) superfine sugar

¼ cup (60 ml) oil

1 cup (235 ml) water

1 teaspoon (5 ml) vanilla extract

1 cup (320 g) low-sugar natural fruit spread

Powdered sugar for dusting (contains cornstarch, use corn-free recipe on page 103)

1. Preheat oven to 350°F (180°C, or gas mark 4).

2. Mix together flour, flax meal, baking powder, sugar, oil, water, and vanilla for about 1 minute or until cake batter reaches a smooth consistency.

3. Divide batter into two foil- or parchment-lined 8-inch (20-cm) round cake pans. Bake for 30 minutes or until center springs back when touched. Let cool in the pans before removing. Peel off parchment or foil. Cool completely.

4. Place one cake on a plate; cover top with fruit spread. Place second cake on top and sprinkle with powdered sugar. Cut into slices.

Yield: 12 slices

Cinnamon Roll Muffins

This quick bread muffin mimics the delicious smells and taste of a cinnamon roll but without a lot of fats and sugars.

For Topping:

1 cup (225 g) brown sugar

½ cup (60 g) rice flour

½ teaspoon (3 g) salt

1 teaspoon (2.3 g) cinnamon

½ cup (112 g) vegetable shortening

For Muffins:

½ cup (100 g) vegetable shortening

½ cup (120 ml) alternative milk beverage

1 cup (200 g) sugar

2 teaspoons (10 ml) vanilla extract

1¾ cup (220 g) rice flour

2 teaspoons (9.2 g) baking powder

1 teaspoon (4.6 g) baking soda

1. Preheat oven to 350°F (180°C, or gas mark 4).

2. To make topping: In a food processor, combine all topping ingredients. Pulse until crumbly. Set aside.

3. To make the muffins: In a mixer, blend together all muffin ingredients until smooth. Grease or line a 12-cup muffin pan with paper liners. Fill cups halfway with batter. Sprinkle with half the topping mixture and then divide remaining batter evenly among muffin cups. Sprinkle the remaining topping mixture over the tops of the muffins. Bake for 30 minutes. Let cool and remove from pan.

Yield: 12 muffins

Millet Molasses Muffins

The millet adds a little crunch to this hearty muffin. Millet is easy to digest and is a good source of Iron. The brown rice flour, ground flaxseeds, millet, and prunes make this muffin a great source of fiber.

½ cup (120 ml) vegetable oil

¼ cup (60 ml) molasses

¼ cup (60 ml) honey

2 cups (250 g) brown rice flour

¼ cup (28 g) ground flax meal

⅓ cup (60 g) millet

1 teaspoon (4.6 g) baking powder

1 teaspoon (4.6 g) baking soda

1 teaspoon (6 g) salt

1 cup (235 ml) alternative milk beverage

½ cup (80 g) raisins or chopped prunes

1. Preheat oven to 350°F (180°C, or gas mark 4).
2. Stir together the oil, molasses, and honey. Add the remaining ingredients and stir until you have a smooth batter. Pour batter into lined or greased muffin pans.
3. Bake for 25 minutes. Cool slightly and remove from pans.

Yield: 16 muffins

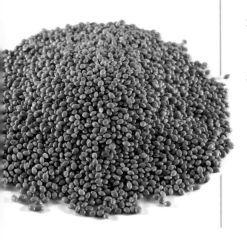

Cinnamon Fritters

For Fritters:

¼ cup (28 g) flax meal

⅔ cup (160 ml) plus 1 table-spoon (15 ml) alternative milk beverage

2 tablespoons (30 ml) vegetable oil

1 tablespoon (13 g) sugar

⅓ cup (42 g) tapioca flour

1⅔ cups (208 g) white or brown rice flour

1 teaspoon (6 g) salt

1 tablespoon (13.8 g) baking powder

½ teaspoon (1.2 g) ground cinnamon

1 cup (150 g) chopped apple

Vegetable oil for frying

For Topping:

1 cup (100 g) powdered sugar (contains corn-starch, use corn-free recipe, right)

1 teaspoon (2.3 g) ground cinnamon

1. In a bowl, mix together all fritter ingredients except oil.

2. Heat oil in a frying pan over medium heat. Place a pea-sized amount of batter in oil; oil is the correct temperature if the batter browns fairly quickly. Lower the heat of the frying pan if necessary.

3. Line a plate with paper towels. With a small ice cream/cookie scoop or a ¼ cup (60 ml) metal measuring cup, drop batter into hot oil. Cook until bottom is golden and then use a metal fork or spatula to flip the fritter over and cook until golden all over.

4. Remove from frying pan and place on a plate to cool. Repeat with remaining batter. (Hint: Cut the first fritter in half to make sure it is cooked all the way through to help you judge the cooking time.)

5. To make the topping: Place either the powdered sugar or the sugar and cinnamon in a bag. Place 2 to 3 fritters in the bag, roll the bag closed, and gently shake to coat. Repeat with remaining fritters. Store fritters in a clean paper bag, sealed.

Yield: 24 fritters

Corn-Free Powdered Sugar Recipe

Powdered sugar contains cornstarch. If you are trying to avoid corn, replace the powdered sugar in the recipes with this corn-free version:

Use a non-contaminated large coffee grinder, ideally one that can hold 1 cup (200 g) or ½ cup (100 g) of sugar at a time. Combine 1 tablespoon (8 g) tapioca or arrow-root starch with 1 cup (200 g) superfine sugar (for smaller amounts, maintain this ratio). Pour into the coffee grinder and grind until you have a very soft, fine powder—the finer the better. Pour into a large resealable plastic bag or sealed glass or stainless steel container. Store in a cool, dark place.

Baby Biscotti

For the teething toddler, make sure you toast the sliced biscotti really well so they are not so crumbly. These are a great source of fiber.

¼ cup (60 ml) olive oil

⅓ cup (70 g) sugar (optional)

⅓ cup (80 ml) honey or molasses

1 teaspoon (5 ml) vanilla extract

2 cups (250 g) rice flour

1½ teaspoons (6.9 g) baking powder

¼ teaspoon (1.1 g) baking soda

¼ teaspoon (1.5 g) salt

1 cup (100 g) certified gluten-free oats, rice bran, or buckwheat flakes

1 cup (110 g) finely shredded carrots

1 cup (70 g) shredded coconut (optional)

½ cup (75 g) raisins, blueberries, dried apricots, or dates

1. Preheat oven to 325°F (170°C, or gas mark 3).
2. Either in a food processor or a mixer, combine oil, sugar, honey, applesauce, and vanilla. Mix well. Add remaining ingredients; mix or process until well combined.
3. On two greased baking sheets, shape dough into four rectangular loaves, two on each baking sheet.
4. Bake for 40 minutes or until golden and firm. Remove from oven and let cool for 10 minutes. With a thin spatula, cut each loaf at an angle into 2-inch (5-cm) strips. Remove each cookie and put cut side down on a new greased baking sheet. Bake for 10 minutes and then flip over and bake for another 10 minutes or until you have reached desired crunchy consistency. If needed, bake 5 minutes more. Cool and store in a covered container for up to 1 week. They freeze well for up to 2 weeks.

Yield: 20 biscotti

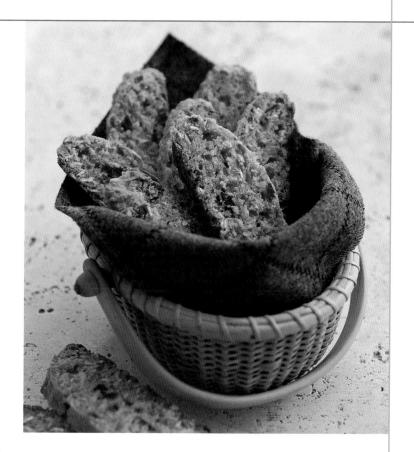

Hidden Gluten Sources

Most parents of children who suffer from a gluten allergy know to avoid wheat, but there are many other sources of gluten that you may use in cooking that you might not even consider. Soy sauce, alcohol, and some teas all contain gluten. Rye, barley, and oats are also off limits to the gluten-free child, although recent studies seem to indicate that certified gluten-free oats may be okay if there is no risk of cross-contamination with wheat in the mills.

Savory Muffins

This is a good muffin together with soups and salads.

    1¾ cups (215 g) brown rice flour

    ¼ cup (28 g) flax meal

    2 tablespoons (25 g) sugar

    2 teaspoons (9.2 g) baking powder

    ¼ teaspoon (1.3 g) baking soda

    ½ teaspoon (0.9 g) dried basil or rosemary

    ½ teaspoon (3 g) salt

    ½ teaspoon (1 g) pepper

    ½ cup (120 ml) alternative milk beverage

    ½ cup (120 ml) tomato sauce

    ⅓ cup (80 ml) olive oil

1. Preheat oven to 350°F (180°C, or gas mark 4).
2. Combine all ingredients in a bowl and whisk together. Pour batter into a greased or paper-lined muffin pan.
3. Bake for 20 minutes or until firm in the center.

Yield: 24 muffins

Sandwich Bread

I am intolerant to yeast, so I have to eat gluten-free tortillas, yeast-free breads, and rice cakes. My kids, however, like their sandwiches.

  1 tablespoon (12 g) active dry yeast

  2 teaspoons (4.7 g) unflavored gelatin

  1 tablespoon (15 ml) honey

  1½ cups (355 ml) warm water

  1 cup (125 g) white rice flour

  ¼ cup (30 g) tapioca flour

  ½ cup (65 g) corn, tapioca, or arrowroot starch

  ¼ cup (28 g) flax meal

  1 teaspoon (6 g) salt

  1½ tablespoons (22 ml) vegetable oil

  1 teaspoon (5 ml) cider vinegar

  Special Equipment: an electric bread machine

1. Combine the yeast, gelatin, and honey in a small bowl. Add the water while gently stirring the yeast mixture. Set aside; mixture should bubble and foam.

2. In a large bowl mix the flours, starch, flax meal, and salt. Stir well.

3. Pour the yeast mixture into the flour blend. Add the oil and vinegar. Stir well and pour the dough into the pan of a bread machine. Follow the manufacturer's directions to bake on the 80-minute setting.

Yield: 1 loaf of bread

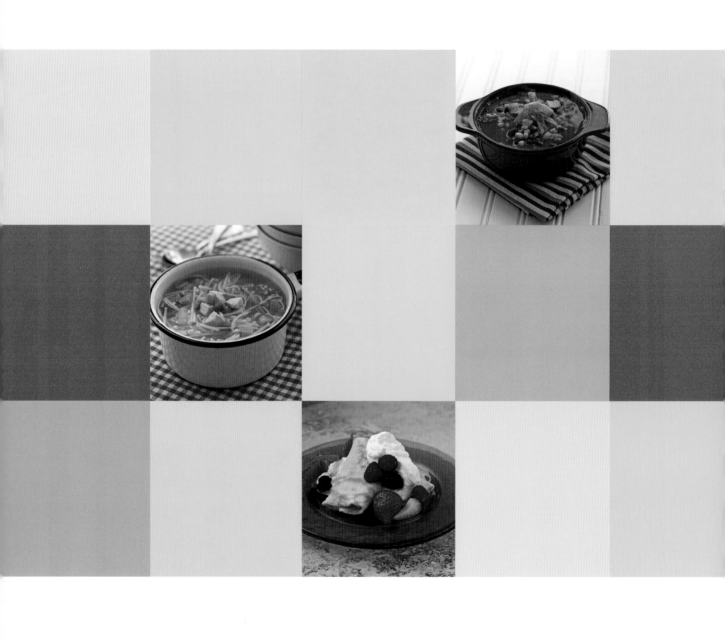

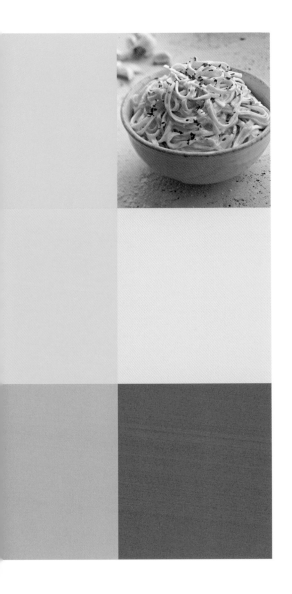

BREAKFAST, LUNCH, and DINNER

Ah! The nutritional mainstay of the day: meals. Part of being a parent is planning healthy meals for your children—a tough task when many of the foods that most people eat are toxic to your family and cause allergic reactions. I've been able to modify my family's favorite recipes to make them allergy-friendly and safe for us to eat. I hope your family enjoys them as well.

"Buttermilk" Pancakes

Variation:
After pouring the batter into the skillet, drop a desired amount of blueberries or chocolate chips onto the uncooked top of the pancake and finish cooking as directed above.

Food Allergies Resource
Interested in reading up about food sensitivity? A good book is *Hidden Food Allergies: Finding the Foods that Cause You Problems and Removing Them from Your Diet* by Stephen Astor, MD (Avery Publishing).

When I surveyed kids about their favorite foods, pancakes ranked high. Enjoy these traditional buttermilk pancakes for breakfast with your wee ones and watch a few cartoons, too. I am always amazed when I make these pancakes. They are so incredibly delicious.

2 cups (250 g) white or brown rice flour

¼ cup (32 g) corn, tapioca, or arrowroot starch

2 tablespoons (25 g) sugar

2 teaspoons (9.2 g) baking powder

1 teaspoon (4.6 g) baking soda

1 teaspoon (6 g) salt

2 cups (475 ml) alternative milk beverage

2 teaspoons (10 ml) vinegar

¼ cup (60 g) vegetable oil

2 teaspoons (10 ml) vanilla extract

1. Combine all ingredients in a large bowl or mixer. Mix batter for 1 minute or until it is smooth.

2. Pour desired amount of batter into a hot greased skillet. When pancake bubbles on top and is lightly golden on the bottom, flip it over with a wide spatula. Cook until golden on bottom and remove to a plate. Repeat with remaining batter. These make great pancake shapes like hearts and letters.

Yield: 10 pancakes

Blue Pancake Crêpes with Blue Applesauce

We call them "blue" pancakes, but sometimes they are purple, which the kids love! These cakes roll nicely. Fill these tasty low-fat rolls with a serving of fruit.

½ cup (75 g) blueberries or blackberries

1 cup (125 g) white or brown rice flour

2 teaspoons (9.2 g) baking powder

¼ teaspoon (1.5 g) salt

¼ cup (28 g) flax meal

¾ cup (175 ml) alternative milk beverage

2 tablespoons (30 ml) oil

2 cups (500 g) Blue Applesauce (see page 19)

1. In a food processor, combine berries, flour, baking powder, salt, flax meal, milk alternative, and oil. Process until smooth.

2. Pour ¼ cup (60 ml) batter into a hot greased skillet, spreading batter thinly around bottom of skillet to make a crêpe. When golden on the bottom, flip and cook on the other side. Remove to a plate and repeat with remaining batter, stacking crêpes as you cook them. Let them cool to room temperature before rolling them. Fill or top with Blue Applesauce and serve with Honey Syrup (recipe follows).

3. You may put waxed paper between crêpes and freeze in a resealable plastic bag for up to 2 weeks. To reheat, toast or microwave them at 30-second intervals.

Yield: about 18 pancakes

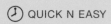

Honey Syrup

Allergies and Asthma Resource
A good place to get literature on allergies and asthma is the Allergy and Asthma Network Mothers of Asthmatics at 800-878-4403 or www.aanma.org.

1 cup (235 ml) water

1 cup (200 g) sugar

Dash cinnamon

¼ cup (60 g) honey

1. In a medium saucepan, combine the water and sugar; bring to a boil over medium-high heat. Stir and cook for 10 minutes or until thickened. Remove from heat and stir in cinnamon and honey. Serve with Blue Pancake Crêpes (see page 111).

Yield: 2¼ cups (760 g)

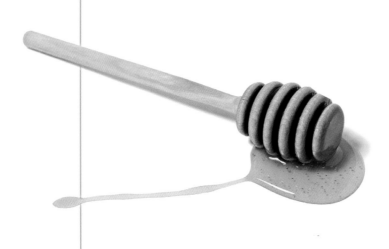

Quick Cinnamon, Apples, and Rice

I make this dish for breakfast, but it makes for a quick snack, or even for a low-sugar treat. It is hearty, healthy, and delicious—and so easy to make!

- 1 large apple, chopped
- ¼ cup (60 ml) vegetable oil
- 1 teaspoon (2.3 g) cinnamon
- 1½ cups (285 g) short-grain brown rice
- ½ cup (115 g) brown sugar, (120 ml) maple syrup, or (120 ml) honey
- 1⅔ cups (400 ml) water

1. Combine all ingredients. Pour into a large saucepan or a rice cooker and cook, covered, according to rice package or rice cooker's directions. Stir once after 10 minutes of cooking and then finish cooking as directed. Enjoy warm or cold.

Yield: 4 servings

Pumpkin Torte

2 tablespoons (14 g) flax meal

1½ cups (355 ml) rice milk or safe milk alternative

2 teaspoons (9.2 g) baking powder

¾ cup (150 g) sugar

⅔ cup (83 g) white or brown rice flour

2 cups (450 g) canned pumpkin

1 teaspoon (5 ml) vanilla extract

½ teaspoon (3 g) salt

2 teaspoons (3.4 g) pumpkin pie spice

¼ cup (25 g) powdered sugar (optional, contains cornstarch, use corn-free recipe on page 103)

1. Preheat oven to 350°F (180°C, or gas mark 4).
2. Place all ingredients except powdered sugar in a blender and purée for about 2 minutes. Pour into a greased 9-inch (23-cm) springform or pie pan.
3. Bake for 35 minutes or until the top and edges are browned and the center is soft but cooked. Let cool. If using a springform pan, remove rim. Slice into wedges. Sprinkle with powdered sugar, if desired.

Yield: 12 slices

Apple Spice French Toast Bake

This is bread pudding, but my girls insist that it tastes like French toast. It's a good source of carbs and fiber for your morning meal.

5 pieces gluten-free bread

1 cup (235 ml) alternative milk beverage or apple juice

½ cup (125 g) applesauce

½ cup (56 g) flax meal

¼ cup (32 g) corn, tapioca, or arrowroot starch

2 teaspoons (10 ml) vegetable oil

½ cup (100 g) sugar

2 teaspoons (4.6 g) vanilla extract

2 teaspoons cinnamon

½ cup (75 g) raisins

1 small apple, chopped

1. Preheat oven to 425°F (220°C, or gas mark 7).

2. Make sure the bread you use is firm and dry (you can either toast it on low heat several times until firm or leave the bread out a few days, loosely covered). Cut bread into small cubes and set aside.

2. Whisk together the remaining ingredients except for the raisins and apple. Grease an 8-inch (20-cm) square baking dish with vegetable oil. Spread the bread cubes evenly in the baking dish and sprinkle with the apple and raisins. Pour the milk mixture over the bread and fruit pieces. Bake, loosely covered with aluminum foil for 35 minutes, or until firm in the center. Let sit 10 minutes before serving. If desired, sprinkle with powdered sugar or cinnamon and sugar. You may spoon additional alternative milk beverage over the top or add a dollop of Rice Dream ice cream (if allowed on your diet) for a special treat.

Yield: 4 servings

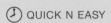

Breakfast Skillet

Corn-Free Variation:
Replace corn tortillas with ½ cup (95 g) cooked quinoa or (110 g) pinto beans.

My children like to tear up the corn tortillas for me. They call this dish the "Messy Breakfast Burrito." It might be messy, but it is a great balanced breakfast to start off the day.

    1 tablespoon (15 ml) olive oil

    1 cup (125 g) chopped squash or potato

    1 small onion, chopped

    3 corn tortillas, torn into 1-inch (2.5-cm) pieces

    1 firm ripe tomato, diced (optional)

    ¼ cup (65 g) salsa

    1 avocado, sliced

1. In a medium skillet with a lid, heat olive oil, squash or potato, and onion. Cook for 1 minute over medium heat. Add tortillas and tomato; cook about 2 minutes longer.

2. Add the salsa and cook, covered, until warmed through. Remove lid and arrange avocado slices over the top. Spoon onto plates and serve.

Yield: 6 servings

Breakfast Patties

My kids love breakfast sausage, but we do not want to chance potential allergens and preservatives in packaged sausage patties. So, we make these instead.

  1 pound (455 g) ground turkey or pork

  2 teaspoons (3 g) poultry seasoning

  ¼ teaspoon (0.6 g) ground nutmeg

  ½ teaspoon (1 g) salt

  ½ teaspoon pepper

  Dash of cloves

  ¼ cup (60 ml) pure maple syrup

  1 small apple, shredded

1. In a large bowl, blend all ingredients together. Form into 12 patties. Coat hands with oil to prevent sticking, if needed.

2. Fry patties in a frying pan over medium heat until thoroughly cooked.

Yield: 12 patties

The Upside of Germs
According to Robert A. Wood, director of the Pediatric Allergy Clinic at Johns Hopkins in Baltimore, "Recent studies indicate that growing up in a large family or a daycare center actually decreases the likelihood of developing an allergy. The fewer germs in terms of infection and the environment, the more time the immune system has to worry about things like allergens."

Low-Sugar Blintzes

These are a delicious treat and are quite easy to prepare. Serve them anytime. You can replace the honey with maple syrup or powdered sugar if you like. Fill with fresh fruit for a low-fat treat.

For Crêpes:

1 cup (235 ml) alternative milk beverage

½ cup (125 g) corn, tapioca, or arrowroot starch

1 cup (125 g) rice flour

1½ tablespoons (22 ml) olive oil

For Filling:

1 tablespoon (15 ml) vegetable oil

2 tablespoons (30 g) packed brown sugar

2 apples, peaches, or bananas, thinly sliced, or 1½ cups (180 g) fresh fruit, such as blueberries, cherries, raspberries, or strawberries

Dash of ground cinnamon (optional)

1. To make the crêpes: In a bowl, mix all crêpe ingredients until smooth. Let sit for 10 minutes.

2. Place a 7-inch (17.5-cm) frying pan (crêpe pan) over medium-high heat and preheat pan until a drop of water sprinkled in the pan immediately evaporates.

3. While swirling the pan around, ladle enough batter into pan to coat with a thin, even crêpe. Cook for about a minute or until it starts to curl on the sides. Flip and cook about 30 seconds more. Repeat with remaining batter. Stack on a plate and cover. Crêpes will become more flexible the longer they sit.

4. To make the filling: In the crêpe pan, cook the oil and brown sugar until melted. Add the fruit and sauté until tender. Stir in the cinnamon, if desired.

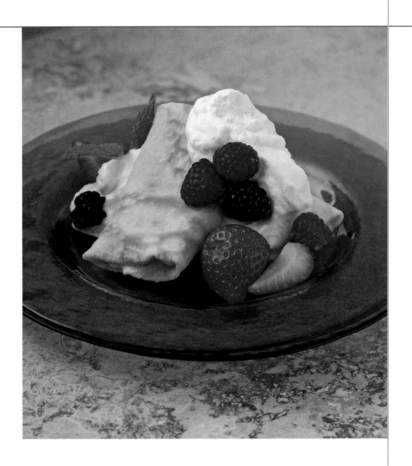

5. To serve, lay a crêpe flat and spoon some filling down the middle. Roll the crêpe around the filling. Top with powdered sugar, reserved filling, and a dollop of Rice Dream ice cream or serve plain.

Yield: 8 blintzes

Scrambled Enchiladas

You can easily cut the recipe in half, if desired.

    8 corn or bean tortillas

    1 tablespoon (15 ml) vegetable oil

    ¼ cup (35 g) diced onion

    ¼ cup (30 g) diced bell pepper

    ½ cup (55 g) diced ham or cooked sausage pieces

    1 cup (260 g) mild enchilada sauce

    ½ cup (130 g) salsa

    2 tablespoons (12 g) sliced scallions

1. Preheat oven to 350°F (180°C, or gas mark 4). Place tortillas in the oven for a few minutes to warm them.

2. Heat oil in a large skillet over medium heat. Add onion and bell pepper; cook for 1 minute. Add the meat and cook 1 minute longer.

3. Remove tortillas from the oven; do not turn off oven. Spoon one-eighth of the meat filling down the center of one tortilla. Roll tortilla up and place seam-side down in an 11 × 7-inch (27.5 × 17.5-cm) baking dish. Repeat with remaining tortillas and meat mixture, setting tortillas side by side in the baking dish.

4. Stir together the enchilada sauce and the salsa. Pour over tortillas. Top with scallions. Return to the oven and cook for 20 minutes. Serve immediately.

Yield: 8 enchiladas

Pastitsio

Often called Greek lasagna, Pastitsio is a baked Greek casserole-like dish. If you opt for the lamb instead of ground beef, add ½ teaspoon (1.2 g) cinnamon for a more ethnic flavor.

1 pound (455 g) ground beef or lamb

½ cup (65 g) onion, chopped

2 teaspoons (5.6 g) garlic, minced

one 25-ounce (690-g) jar pasta sauce

1¾ cups (425 ml) alternative milk beverage

3 tablespoons (24 g) corn, tapioca, or arrowroot starch

one 13-ounce (370-g) box elbow macaroni, cooked and drained

Salt and pepper

1. Preheat oven to 350°F (180°C, or gas mark 4).

2. In a large skillet cook meat, onion, and garlic until meat is brown. Drain fat. Stir in pasta sauce and simmer.

3. In a saucepan add the milk alternative and starch and cook for 3 minutes, or until thick and bubbly, stirring frequently. Remove from heat. Add salt and pepper to taste. Pour 1 cup (235 ml) of milk mixture into a bowl and set aside. Pour the remaining milk sauce over the cooked noodles and mix until well coated.

4. In an 8 × 8 × 2-inch (20 × 20 × 5-cm) greased baking dish, layer half of the noodle mixture, all of the meat mixture, and the remaining noodle mixture. Pour reserved milk mixture over the top. Bake for 40 minutes. Let stand 10 minutes before serving.

Yield: 8 servings

Variation:
Sauté 2 cups (300 grams) of vegetables and use in place of

Celebrities Have Food Allergies Too!
Are your kids are feeling different from their peers because of their diet? Remind them that there are plenty of famous people who have dietary restrictions as well. Former Spice Girl Geri Halliwell follows a strict dairy- and wheat-free diet. Orlando Bloom has an intolerance to dairy. And Alicia Silverstone, Casey Affleck, Natalie Portman, Moby, Prince, and designer Stella McCartney are vocal vegans.

Butternut Squash Risotto Bake

Stress and Allergies

Try to alleviate stress in your life and the lives of your children—especially your children with food allergies. Researchers know that stress plays a major role in allergies by upsetting digestion, suppressing immunity, and weakening adrenal response.

The origins of butternut squash are Mexico and Central America. This wonderful food deserves a place on the table for anyone wanting to boost intake of health-building vitamins A and C.

4 cups (940 ml) water, divided

3 bouillon cubes

2 teaspoons (10 ml) olive oil

1 small zucchini, shredded

2 cups (280 g) peeled and cubed butternut squash

1 small onion, chopped

1½ cups (300 g) arborio rice or short-grain brown rice

Salt and pepper

1. Preheat oven to 425°F (220°C, or gas mark 7).

2. In a bowl, place 1 cup (235 ml) warm water and bouillon cubes; stir until dissolved.

3. In a medium saucepan over medium-high heat, add oil, zucchini, squash, and onion. Cook for four minutes. Add rice and sauté for four minutes more. Add the bouillon liquid. Cook, stirring, until almost all liquid is absorbed. Add the remaining 3 cups (705 ml) of water. Cover saucepan and let cook until squash is tender and falling apart, about 25 minutes.

4. Spoon mixture into a greased baking dish and bake for 20 minutes. Cut into squares and serve.

Yield: 10 servings

The Very Best Spaghetti

Rice noodles are delicate, but with the right attention they can be perfect. Two boxes of noodles will feed a hungry family of four to five. Different brands of noodles cook differently, but my advice for any gluten-free noodle is to cook it in a lot of water! 8 cups (1.8 liters) water!

1 teaspoon (6 g) salt

Dash olive oil

two 8 ounce (225 g) boxes of spaghetti rice noodles

one 25 ounce (710 g) jar of your favorite allergy-friendly spaghetti sauce

1 pound (455 g) sautéed vegetables and/or cooked meat

Fresh chopped herbs for sprinkling

1. Bring water to a boil in a large pot. Add salt and oil.

2. When water comes to a rolling boil, add the two boxes of spaghetti. With a wooden spoon, give the noodles a stir to prevent sticking. Turn down the heat to medium. Leaving pot uncovered, stir frequently to ensure even cooking. Follow package directions for cooking times. When noodles are at desired consistency, remove from heat and pour into a strainer. With a wooden spoon, gently stir and lift noodles while running them under cool water. After rinsing them they will feel firmer and less sticky. Shake strainer gently to discard any excess water. Place noodles on a large plate.

3. Combine spaghetti sauce and sautéed vegetables or meat in a large saucepan over medium-high heat and bring to a full boil. Pour sauce over noodles, tossing to coat well. You may keep the plate in a warm oven until ready to serve (no more than 20 minutes). Sprinkle with herbs.

Yield: 5 servings

Variation:
For those little ones who prefer plain noodles, after rinsing with cool water, rinse with warm water. Toss with olive oil and cooked vegetables.

Fettuccine Alfredo

Variation:
Sauté strips of cooked chicken in garlic and olive oil. Place over noodles and sauce.

Rich and filling, this Alfredo is comforting on a cold night. Add some protein and vegetables for a complete healthy meal.

two 8-ounce (225-g) boxes fettuccine or penne pasta

2 tablespoons (30 ml) olive oil

1 teaspoon (2.8 g) or desired amount of fresh chopped garlic

1 cup (235 ml) alternative milk beverage

4 teaspoons (10.5 g) corn, tapioca, or arrowroot starch

¼ cup (15 g) chopped fresh parsley

1. Cook noodles according to package directions, stirring frequently to ensure even cooking. Strain noodles and rinse with cold water.
2. While noodles are cooking, heat the oil in a saucepan and sauté the garlic. In a large bowl, whisk together the milk alternative and starch. Pour into the saucepan with the sautéed garlic and oil; bring to a boil over medium heat until thickened.
3. Rinse noodles with hot water and strain into a bowl. Pour warm sauce over noodles. Sprinkle with parsley or chives.

Yield: 5 servings

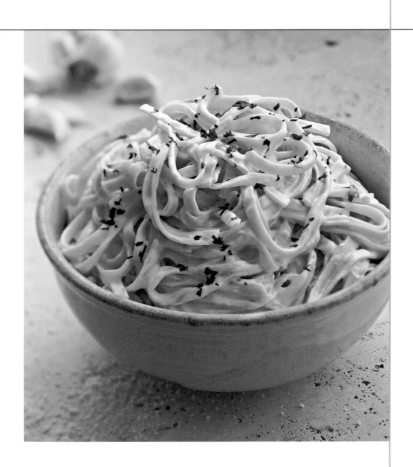

Quinoa Stew

Preparing Quinoa

Quinoa is coated with a natural substance called saponin that protects the grain by repelling insects and birds. Rinsing the quinoa is important to avoid a raw or bitter taste. You can tell if there is saponin if you see soapy looking "suds" when you swish the grains in water. Keep rinsing until the suds disappear to make the grain more palatable to young palates.

Omit the steak in this unique and hearty dish to make it vegan.

1 cup (170 g) quinoa

2½ cups (570 ml) vegetable broth or water, divided

½ pound (225 g) cubed steak (optional)

2 tablespoons (30 ml) olive oil, divided

½ cup (80 g) sweet onion, diced

1 teaspoon (2.8 g) minced garlic

1 cup (160 g) baby carrots

1 cup (100 g) chopped celery stalk

1 zucchini, cubed

1 cup (70 g) mushrooms, chopped or sliced

1 can (16 ounces or 454 g) stewed tomatoes, not drained

1 teaspoon (2.5 g) cumin (optional)

1 teaspoon (2.5 g) chili powder or (1.8 g) oregano

Salt and pepper to taste

1. Rinse quinoa in a strainer with cold water. Place rinsed quinoa and 1 cup (235 ml) broth or water in a saucepan and cook, covered, on medium-low heat for 15 minutes or until soft.

2. In a skillet, sauté the steak with 1 tablespoon (15 ml) olive oil until browned. Set aside.

3. Heat the remaining 1 tablespoon (15 ml) olive oil in a large soup pot and sauté the onions and garlic over medium heat for 5 minutes. Add celery and carrots to the soup pot and cook an additional 5 minutes, stirring often.

4. Add the zucchini, mushrooms, tomatoes, and remaining 1½ cups (355 ml) water or vegetable broth to soup pot. Stir in cumin, if using, and chili powder or oregano. Simmer, covered, for 10 to 15 minutes or until vegetables are tender. Stir in cooked quinoa, steak, and salt and pepper to taste.

Yield: 4 servings

From-Scratch Mac-n-Cheese

Serve this hearty mac-n-cheese with roasted chicken or chops. Meals from scratch always taste better and are better for you. The cooked carrots deliver the color to noodles and add nutrients.

1 cup (235 ml) alternative milk beverage

2 tablespoons (30 ml) plus 1 teaspoon (5 ml) vegetable oil, divided

4 teaspoons (10.5 g) corn, tapioca, or arrowroot starch

1 cup (130 g) carrots, cooked and mashed

2 cups (280 g) cooked, cooled gluten-free elbow macaroni

Salt and pepper

1. Whisk together the milk alternative, 2 tablespoons (30 ml) oil, and starch in a large saucepan; bring to a boil over medium heat. Reduce heat to low, stir in the mashed carrots and remaining 1 teaspoon oil. Add the macaroni and stir until heated thoroughly. Sprinkle with salt and pepper to taste.

Yield: 4 servings

Variation:
For Confetti Macaroni, add 1 cup (125 grams) diced chicken, ham, or drained albacore tuna, and 1 cup (125 grams) assorted vegetables like peas or broccoli. Add with the macaroni and stir until heated through.

Video Resource for Dietary Restrictions
Have you or your child been recently diagnosed with food restrictions or are you looking for more information? A new video program series on DVD is the perfect resource to give to your child's teacher or health care provider to help them work with your child to handle and understand the diagnosis. Go online to www.newer-aprodutions.com or call 866-963-9372.

Red Sauce

Low-sugar variation:
Omit sugar.

Choosing Cooking Oils

Oils are commonly derived from allergenic foods like peanuts and soybeans. Be careful in choosing the type of oil you use and how it is refined. Generally, highly refined oils—even peanut oil—can be safe. Less highly refined oils, including cold-pressed oils, may not always prove safe. And always avoid using oils that have been used for frying because cross-contamination can occur.

If you have kids who won't eat anything with onions in it, simply process all the ingredients in a food processor until smooth. Place in a saucepan and cook as directed. Use all organic ingredients for a healthier touch.

1 tablespoon (15 ml) oil

½ white onion, finely chopped, or 1 table spoon (5 g) dehydrated onion

1 can (6 ounces or 170 g) Italian-style tomato paste

2 teaspoons (8.4 g) sugar

1 teaspoon (1.8 g) dried basil

1 teaspoon (2.8 g) fresh, minced, or powdered garlic

Splash of gluten-free red wine

1. Heat the oil in a medium saucepan over medium-high heat; sauté onion. Add the tomato paste plus 1 can (6 ounces) of water and stir until combined. Add the rest of the ingredients and cook over medium heat until bubbly, stirring occasionally. Add more water if needed. Remove from heat and pour over pizza crust.

Yield: enough for one pizza

Pizza Stuffed Mushrooms

This recipe gives you all the great pizza flavor without any of the crust. Eating these treats is like popping pizza bites. This is also a great dish for moms who are watching their calories—a few of these pizza bites cures the desire to turn to greasy pizza!

12 small portobello or 24 small white mushrooms

½ cup (60 g) coarsely chopped pepperoni

1 cup (260 g) pizza sauce

1 zucchini, diced

⅓ cup (40 g) bell pepper, diced

¼ cup (35 g) onion, chopped

2 tablespoons fresh or dried (5.3 g or 9 g) chopped basil
    or (7.6 g) or 2.6 g) parsley

1. Preheat oven to 350°F (180°C, or gas mark 4).
2. Clean mushrooms and remove stems. On a lightly greased baking sheet, place mushrooms open side up. Spray with cooking oil spray.
3. In a bowl, mix together pepperoni, pizza sauce, zucchini, bell pepper, and onion. Spoon mixture into each mushroom. Sprinkle with basil or parsley. Bake for 20 minutes. Serve immediately.

Yield: 12 (or 24 small) stuffed mushrooms

Variation:
You can stuff many different kinds of vegetables. Cut a zucchini in half lengthwise and hollow it out to stuff. Cored and seeded bell peppers also work nicely.

Learn How to Read Labels
Basically, the ingredients statements on packaged foods are complete and accurate. Part of the task, however, is recognizing the terms on the ingredient label that indicate offending foods. For example, for milk intolerances, look for caseinate, whey, and lactose. Want help identifying those items that you or your child needs to avoid? Contact the Food Allergy and Anaphylaxis Network (www.foodallergy.org) for label-reading cards that can help you recognize the terms to avoid.

Pizza Noodles

Who says pizza isn't good for you? This dish gives you the flavors of pizza without all the greasy fat! To lower the fat content further, use low-fat turkey pepperoni and lean ground turkey and increase the veggies by adding bell peppers, onions, broccoli, and spinach.

two 8-ounce (225-g) boxes of your favorite gluten-free noodle shape

1 pound (455 g) ground beef, pork, or turkey

one 10-ounce (280-g) jar pizza or marinara sauce

⅓ cup (40 g) chopped pepperoni

1 cup (70 g) sliced mushrooms

2 tablespoons (17 g) chopped olives

Splash of gluten-free red wine (optional)

2 tablespoons chopped fresh (7.6 g) or dried (2.6 g) parsley

1. Preheat oven to 425°F (220°C, or gas mark 7).

2. Cook noodles according to package directions but remove them a few minutes before they are done; they should feel al dente. Rinse with cold water and set aside.

3. In a large skillet, brown meat until no longer pink in the middle. Add sauce, pepperoni, mushrooms, and olives. Add a splash of wine, if desired. Cook until bubbly. Remove from heat.

4. Add noodles to the sauce mixture and gently stir. Gently pour into a 9 × 13-inch (22.5 × 32.5-cm) casserole dish. Top with parsley. Bake for 15 minutes or until sauce is bubbly.

Yield: 6 servings

Variation:
For Pizza Rice, replace the noodles with 2 cups (330 g) cooked rice. Add to sauce and bake as directed.

Avoid the Pitfalls of Eating Out
Although cooking for your child is the best way to go, sometimes it can't be avoided—you end up in a restaurant. Foods are not labeled in food-service operations, so you must ask the server, manager, or cook about ingredients. Unfortunately, cross-contamination can occur easily in a restaurant and accounts for some inadvertent food-allergy deaths. You can get information about eating out safely by going to www.glutenfreepassport.com.

Pizza Dough

In a world where all the pizza is made with wheat flour, your family will love this alternative pizza dough that won't cause any allergic reactions.

1 tablespoon (12 g) active yeast

⅔ cup (80 g) white or brown rice flour

½ cup (60 g) tapioca flour

2 tablespoons (16 g) corn, tapioca, or arrowroot starch

½ teaspoon (3 g) salt

1 tablespoon (7 g) unflavored gelatin

1 teaspoon (1.4 g) dried basil

⅔ cup (160 ml) warm water

1 tablespoon (13 g) sugar

1 teaspoon (4.5 ml) olive oil

1 teaspoon (5ml) cider vinegar

1. Preheat oven to 425°F (220°C, or gas mark 7).

2. In a mixer, blend all ingredients on low speed. Scrape sides down. Beat on high speed for 3 minutes. Liberally sprinkle rice flour on dough and then press dough into a lightly greased 12-inch (30-cm) pizza pan, continuing to sprinkle with flour to prevent sticking to hands.

4. Bake pizza crust for 20 minutes. Remove from oven. Spread pizza crust with your favorite sauce and toppings. Bake with toppings for an additional 20 minutes or until top is nicely browned.

Yield: 1 pizza crust

Look out for Lecithin
Lecithin can be made from either soybean or egg and can contain protein residues, so be sure to look for it on labels and avoid it if you have a soy or egg allergy.

Chili-Mac

Keep in Mind

Buy organic when you can to avoid pesticide residues. For your meats, seek out organic, free range, no nitrates, and antibiotic-free varieties. Look for organic, sulfite-free dried fruits. Purchase certified gluten-free grains. Always read your labels and call the manufacturer to check about possible contamination. And finally, remember that a happy baker's food tastes better, so stay positive!

Don't plan on serving leftovers for lunch the next day; there are never leftovers of this wholesome dish in my house.

- 1 box (8 to 12 ounces or 225 to 340 g) gluten-free elbow macaroni
- 1 pound (455 g) ground beef
- ¾ cup (95 g) chopped onion
- 1 can (8 ounces or 225 g) tomato paste
- 1 can (4 ounces or 115 g) diced green chili peppers, drained
- 2 teaspoons (5.2 g) chili powder
- ½ teaspoon (3 g) salt
- 1 teaspoon (2.8 g) minced garlic
- 1 can (15 ounces, or 420 g) red kidney beans, drained

1. Cook noodles according to the package directions. Rinse with cold water and set aside.
2. In a skillet, brown beef and onion until cooked completely. Stir in the tomato paste plus one can (8 ounces) of water. Add the chili peppers, chili powder, salt, and garlic. Add the noodles and the kidney beans and stir to combine.

Yield: 5 servings

Sloppy Joe Potato Skillet

Omit the potatoes and serve this in your favorite gluten-free rolls.

   1 pound (455 g) ground beef or turkey

   2 medium potatoes, chopped

   1 onion, chopped

   one 15½-ounce (430-g) can Hunts Manwich Original Sloppy
      Joe sauce (gluten-free)

   ½ cup (120 ml) water

1. Brown meat, potatoes, and onion in a skillet. Pour in the sauce
   and the water. Cover and simmer for 30 minutes or until potatoes
   are tender.

Yield: 5 servings

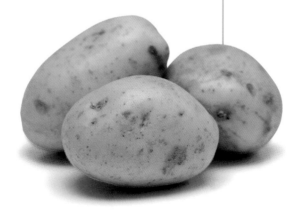

Grandma's Tamale Casserole

Heredity and Allergies

Allergies are genetic, making them much more likely to develop in children born to parents who suffer with either food or environmental allergies. The interesting part is this: The nature of the allergy that the child develops is not genetically controlled. For example, let's say that a child is born to parents who suffer from pollen allergies. One would think that the child would then develop pollen allergies, right? Perhaps, but the child may instead experience food allergies.

My grandma used to make this. When she gave me this recipe, I couldn't believe how easy it is to prepare.

- 2 tablespoons (30 ml) oil
- 1 pound (455 g) ground beef or turkey
- 1 cup (160 g) chopped onions
- ⅛ teaspoon (0.4 g) garlic powder
- 1 teaspoon (6 g) salt
- 2 teaspoons (5.2 g) chili powder
- 2 cans (8 ounces, or 225 g) tomato sauce
- ½ cup (30 grams) parsley
- 1 can (15 ounces or 420 g) pitted ripe olives, drained
- 1 beef bouillon cube
- 1 cup (235 ml) warm water

1. Preheat oven to 350°F (180°C, or gas mark 4).
2. Heat oil in a large skillet over medium heat and brown beef or turkey. Add onions and the next six ingredients (through olives). Place the bouillon cube in the warm water and stir until dissolved. Stir into meat mixture and bring to a boil.
3. Pour mixture into a 12-ounce (355 ml) baking dish. Bake for 30 minutes. Let sit for 5 minutes before serving.

Yield: 8 servings

Vegetarian Tamale Casserole

I took my Grandma's Tamale Casserole recipe and lowered the fat. You still get the same great taste and a little more color!

1 cup (235 ml) water

1 vegetable bouillon cube

2 cans (8 ounces or 225 g) tomato paste

1 can (15 ounces or 420 g) Mexican-seasoned pinquito beans

½ cup (60 g) red bell pepper, chopped

½ cup (60 g) green bell pepper, chopped

2 teaspoons (5.6 g) minced garlic

½ cup (30 g) chopped cilantro, divided

¼ cup (30 g) chopped olives

1 ripe tomato, chopped

1 zucchini, chopped

2 tablespoons (12 g) chopped scallions

2 teaspoons (5.2 g) chili powder

1. Preheat oven to 425°F (220°C, or gas mark 7).

2. Heat water in a saucepan. Add the bouillon cube; stir until dissolved. Add the tomato paste plus one can (8 ounces) of water. Stir in the beans, bell peppers, garlic, ¼ cup (15 g) cilantro, olives, tomato, zucchini, scallions, and the chili powder.

3. Pour mixture into a 9 × 13-inch (23 × 33-cm) baking dish. Top with the remaining ¼ cup (15 g) cilantro. Bake for 25 minutes. Let sit for 5 minutes and serve.

Yield: 8 servings

Alli's Noodles

Lactose Intolerance

Lactose intolerance is a funny thing. Some people with lactose intolerance can actually handle milk products in small doses. It's up to each individual to determine how much is okay. While one person may be able to have a bowl of ice cream without any reaction, another may experience a problem while eating a food contaminated with a small amount of dairy.

My daughter Allison loves this noodle dish. All the vegetables make it attractive, and it's a good, simple allergy-safe dish to bring to potlucks.

1 box (8 to 12 ounces or 225 to 340 g) favorite gluten-free noodle shapes

1 tablespoon (15 ml) olive oil, plus more for drizzling

1 cup (70 g) mushrooms, sliced

1 cup (150 g) mixed red, yellow, and green bell peppers, sliced

2 teaspoons (5.6 g) garlic

½ onion, sliced

1 cup (150 g) cherry tomatoes

2 teaspoons (1.8 g) fresh basil, chopped

Salt and pepper

1. Cook noodles according to package directions; drain and rinse.

2. In a frying pan, heat 1 tablespoon (15 ml) olive oil over medium-high heat and sauté the mushrooms, bell peppers, garlic, and onion for 5 minutes or until cooked but still crunchy.

3. In a large bowl, combine the warm noodles, sautéed vegetables and their juices, cherry tomatoes, and fresh basil. Drizzle with olive oil to coat well. Season to taste with salt and pepper.

Yield: 8 servings

Tortilla-less Enchiladas

Impress your guests with this beautiful dish.

1 teaspoon (5 ml) oil

1 cup (120 g) chopped zucchini

1 cup (120 g) chopped red pepper

1 cup (120 g) chopped red onion

1 can (4 ounces or 115 g) diced green chiles, undrained

1 pound (455 g) ground chicken or beef

1 cup (225 g) salsa

1 can (15 ounces or 420 g) refried beans

1½ cups (390 g) mild green or red enchilada sauce

¼ cup (25 g) each of chopped scallions, tomatoes, and cilantro

1. Preheat oven to 375°F (190°C, or gas mark 5).

2. Heat oil in a large skillet over medium-high heat; cook the zucchini, red pepper, and onion for 3 minutes. Add chiles. Set aside.

3. In a frying pan, cook ground meat until browned. Stir in salsa; set aside.

4. Grease a 9-inch (23-cm) round baking pan. Spread the refried beans in the pan, top with vegetables, then meat. Pour enchilada sauce over the top. Sprinkle with scallions.

5. Bake for 40 minutes. Let cool 10 minutes before serving.

Yield: 8 servings

Turkey Rice Pie

Add a salad to this main dish for a light summer dinner.

        1 cup (235 ml) alternative milk beverage

        1 tablespoon (8 g) corn, tapioca, or arrowroot starch

        ½ teaspoon (3 g) salt

        1½ cups (250 g) cooked white rice

        1 cup (225 g) cooked turkey coarsely chopped

        1 cup (30 g) chopped fresh spinach

        1 teaspoon (2.8 g) minced garlic

        ¼ cup (25 g) sliced scallions

1. Preheat oven to 325°F (170°C, or gas mark 3).
2. Grease a 9-inch (22.5-cm) glass pie plate.
3. In a bowl, stir together milk alternative, starch, and salt. Add the rice, turkey, spinach, garlic, and scallions. Pour into the prepared pie dish. Bake for 45 minutes or until a knife inserted in the center comes out clean. Remove and let sit 10 minutes before serving.

Yield: 6 slices

Broccoli Beef Noodles

4 teaspoons (20 ml) vegetable oil, divided

1 cup (175 g) sliced fajita meat

2 teaspoons (10 ml) molasses

2 tablespoons (30 ml) gluten-free tamari

2 teaspoons (5.5 g) grated fresh ginger

1 beef bouillon cube

1 tablespoon (8 g) corn, tapioca, and arrowroot starch

1 cup (235 ml) warm water

1 cup (90 g) sliced broccoli

2 cups (280 g) cooked gluten-free spaghetti

¼ cup (25 g) sliced scallions

1. In a skillet over medium-high heat, add 2 teaspoons (10 ml) vegetable oil and the meat. Sauté until fully cooked. Add the molasses, tamari, and ginger. Coat the meat. Add the bouillon cube and cornstarch to the water and stir until dissolved. Add the broccoli to the meat mixture and stir to coat. Add the water mixture. Let cook until thickened.

2. Add the spaghetti, scallions, and remaining vegetable oil. Cook until heated. Serve.

Yield: 6 servings

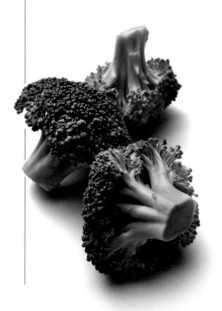

Chicken Nuggets

Preventing Food Allergies
One way food allergy specialists say you can reduce your child's susceptibility to food allergies is to begin while you're pregnant. Women should avoid peanuts, tree nuts, and shellfish while pregnant and also while breastfeeding. Then avoid giving a baby cow's milk or other dairy products until the child's first birthday. Don't introduce eggs until eighteen to twenty-four months. Finally, to safeguard against the child's having a reaction to peanuts, wait until a child is three to give them to him or her.

So simple and delicious, you will never miss your nuggets again! You can even freeze these for a quick lunch—just like the real deal but healthier and better tasting.

- 1 pound (455 g) chicken breast, cut into chunks
- 2 tablespoons (30 ml) vegetable oil
- 2 teaspoons (10 ml) gluten-free tamari
- 1 teaspoon (6 g) salt
- 1 teaspoon (4.2 g) sugar
- ½ teaspoon (0.8 g) poultry seasoning
- ¼ teaspoon (0.5 g) black pepper
- ¼ teaspoon (0.7 g) garlic powder
- ¼ cup (60 ml) water
- ½ cup (60 g) rice flour
- ¼ cup (30 g) corn, tapioca, or arrowroot starch
- ½ teaspoon (2.3 g) baking soda
- Vegetable oil for frying

1. Wash cut chicken in cold water. Mix together 2 tablespoons (30 ml) oil, tamari, salt, sugar, poultry seasoning, pepper, and garlic powder in a large resealable plastic freezer bag. Place chicken into bag and shake, coating each piece.

2. Place bag into freezer for about 30 minutes. Remove from freezer and pour the water into the bag; shake again.

3. In a bowl, mix the flour, cornstarch, and baking soda. Pour into the bag with the chicken. Shake again to coat.

4. In a hot frying pan with 1 inch (2.5 cm) of oil, place a few nuggets at a time and fry until golden brown on both sides, about 3 minutes per side. Remove to a plate lined with paper towels to drain. Repeat with remaining nuggets. Serve with Sweet Dipping Sauce (page 141).

5. To store, let nuggets cool to room temperature. Place in a heavy-duty resealable plastic freezer bag. Try to press as much air as possible out of the bag before placing in the freezer. Can be kept frozen up to 3 weeks. To heat frozen nuggets, place in a 350°F (180°C, or gas mark 4) oven for 10 minutes or microwave until hot.

Yield: 10 servings

Sweet Dipping Sauce

🕐 QUICK N EASY

½ cup (125 g) Dijon or honey mustard

3 tablespoons (45 ml) rice vinegar

¼ cup (60 ml) olive oil

½ cup (170 g) honey

1 tablespoon (15 g) brown sugar (optional)

1. Whisk all ingredients in a bowl. Serve with nuggets. Store in the refrigerator, covered, for up to 4 days.

Yield: 1½ cup (360 g)

Hot Dog, Bean, and Tortilla Casserole

Allergy-Friendly Meats

There are many organic meat products that now cater to gluten-free and dairy-free diets. Try looking at your local natural food store or order online at retailers like www. organicprairie.com.

11 corn tortillas

11 chicken hot dogs

one 15-ounce (420-g) can Mexican-seasoned beans or barbeque beans

2 cups (520 g) purchased salsa

1. Preheat oven to 350°F (180°C, or gas mark 4).

2. Take a few tortillas at a time, sprinkle them with water, and microwave for 30 seconds or until soft. Repeat with remaining tortillas. Set aside, covered.

3. In each tortilla place 1 hot dog and add 3 tablespoons beans. Roll up and place seam-side down next to each other in a greased 9 × 13-inch (23 × 33-cm) pan. Pour salsa over entire dish. Bake for 20 minutes.

Yield: 11 servings

Stick Dogs

With or without the sticks, these are just as good as the store-bought ones, but if you make them yourself you can use nitrate-free, free-range hot dogs and use organic ingredients. Who would have thought corn dogs could be healthy?

10 gluten- and sulfite-free hot dogs

1 cup (125 g) millet flour

½ cup (56 g) flax meal

⅓ cup (115 g) honey or sugar

1½ teaspoons (6.9 g) baking powder

½ teaspoon (1.2 g) dry mustard

1 cup (235 ml) alternative milk beverage or water

½ cup (120 ml) olive or vegetable oil, divided

1. Rinse hot dogs with water and pat dry.

2. In a medium-size bowl, mix together the flour, flax meal, honey, baking powder, dry mustard, milk alternative, and 2 tablespoons (30 ml) oil.

3. Heat the remaining oil in a frying pan until hot. Dip a hot dog into the batter and coat well. Shake off excess. Fry two hot dogs at a time and cook until golden. Remove to a paper towel-lined plate and drain. Serve with your favorite allergy-safe hot dog dips.

4. To freeze, let stick dogs come to room temperature. Wrap in foil or waxed paper and place in a heavy-duty resealable plastic freezer bag. Freeze for up to 1 month.

Yield: 10 stick dogs

Variation:
For mini dogs, cut each hot dog into 3 pieces. Coat with batter and fry until golden.

Kid-Approved Allergy-Friendly Foods
In a hurry and need a quick, frozen, kid-friendly food? Try Ian's Natural Foods—they make great-tasting real chicken nuggets and turkey corndogs. They are available in many grocery stores.

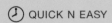

Ranch Dressing

Lactose Intolerance or Milk Allergy?

Lactose intolerance and milk allergies are not the same thing! Those with lactose intolerance lack the enzyme necessary to digest lactose (milk sugar) and should substitute dairy with products made from soy, rice, certified gluten-free oats, grains, or nuts. Those with milk allergies react to the proteins found in milk and should avoid products with casein milk protein, such as many dairy-free cheeses.

1 cup (240 g) Mock Mayonnaise (see recipe page 163)

1 tablespoon (10 g) minced onion

2 tablespoons (6 g) minced chives or scallions

1 teaspoon (2.8 g) garlic powder

1 tablespoon (4 g) chopped parsley

¼ teaspoon (1.5 g) salt

¼ teaspoon (0.5 g) pepper

Squeeze of lemon juice

1. Whisk all ingredients in a bowl. Stir in additional lemon juice or water to reach desired consistency. Chill in a resealable container until ready to serve. Use within 3 days.

Yield: about 1¼ cup (260 g)

Salsa Vinaigrette

🕐 QUICK N EASY

½ cup (130 grams) purchased salsa

¼ cup (60 ml) olive oil

¼ cup (60 ml) rice vinegar

1. Whisk all ingredients together and serve. Store for 1 week in the refrigerator.

Yield: about 1 cup (235 g)

Honey Mustard Dressing

🕐 QUICK N EASY

¼ cup (60 ml) olive oil

¼ cup (60 ml) rice vinegar

3 basil leaves, cleaned

1 tablespoon (15 g) Dijon mustard

1 tablespoon (20 g) honey

Dash gluten-free wine

Salt and pepper

1. Place all ingredients in a food processor. Pulse until smooth. Serve immediately.

Yield: a little over ½ cup (120 g)

Happy Burgers

What to Do after a Food Allergy Diagnosis

Once a food allergy has been diagnosed, there are several key things that you should do to avoid your child's suffering in the future. They are as follows:

Read labels—Make sure you avoid all products with the allergen.

Prep for an emergency— Have antihistamines or prescribed medications on hand in case your child mistakenly eats a toxic food.

Tell everyone—Inform the sitter, Grandma and Grandpa, and playmates' parents; explain that your child must eat only food given by you or approved by you.

Give your kids the fun of quick foods without the fats and preservatives. Whenever your child wants a fast food burger meal, make this burger, wrap it in waxed paper, and serve it with frozen gluten-free french fries and soda or a smoothie! I have even gone as far as purchasing the toy and a soda from a fast food restaurant and serving them along with this meal in the restaurant's kid's meals bag (ask for the toy to be inside a meal bag).

1 pound (455 g) ground beef or turkey

1 teaspoon (5 ml) gluten-free tamari

½ teaspoon (1.4 g) garlic powder

½ teaspoon (1.2 g) onion powder

Salt and pepper

½ cup (120 g) Mock Mayonnaise (see recipe page 163)

¼ cup (60 g) ketchup

1 teaspoon (5 g) mustard

2 teaspoons (10 g) sweet or dill relish

5 to 6 whole lettuce leaves, washed and dried (I prefer iceberg.)

1. In a medium bowl mash together first 4 ingredients (through onion powder) with a fork. Form patties, season with salt and pepper, and fry in a skillet until no longer pink in the middle.

2. In a small bowl mix together the mock mayonnaise, ketchup, mustard, and relish.

3. Place a piece of waxed paper on a flat surface. Put a piece of lettuce with the curved side up, like a bowl, on the paper. Place a hot beef patty in the center. Spoon on desired amount of sauce. Fold 2 opposite sides of the lettuce over the meat. Fold next 2 sides over. Wrap in waxed paper. Serve as directed above.

Yield: 6 burgers

Veggie Burger

I get tired of eating meat, but I need something hearty and healthy to feed to my family. This is an alternative that my family enjoys, and it provides a serving of veggies and grains in one patty.

1 cup (225 g) canned cannellini beans, drained and rinsed

1 cup (170 g) cooked quinoa or brown rice, firmly packed

3 cloves garlic, minced finely

1 cup (120 g) grated carrot

1 tablespoon (8 g) corn, tapioca, or arrowroot starch

½ teaspoon (1.5 g) garlic salt

¼ cup (28 g) flax meal

½ cup (60 g) certified gluten-free oat flour or brown rice flour

Ground black pepper to taste

¼ cup (60 ml) light olive oil or canola oil, for frying

Additional flour for rolling

1. In a food processor, purée beans until smooth. Add remaining ingredients except oil and pulse until mixture is moist but not smooth.

2. In a frying pan, heat oil over medium-high heat. Sprinkle additional flour on a plate. Form the bean mixture into hamburger-sized patties. Dip each patty in flour, coating both sides.

3. Cook one patty at a time in oil for 3 to 5 minutes on each side. Drain on a plate lined with paper towels. Serve immediately.

Yield: 6 burgers

Allergy-Friendly Vegetarian Foods

It can be difficult to be a vegetarian when you have food allergies. Many vegetarian products contain gluten, dairy, and soy. But have hope—more and more companies offer allergy-friendly foods. Try Garden Burgers at your local grocery store or from www.gardenburger.com. They offer gluten-free Black Bean Chipotle and Flame Grilled burgers and a Veggie Breakfast Sausage. Looking for soy-free foods? Try the Garden Vegan and Sun-Dried Tomato Basil burgers!

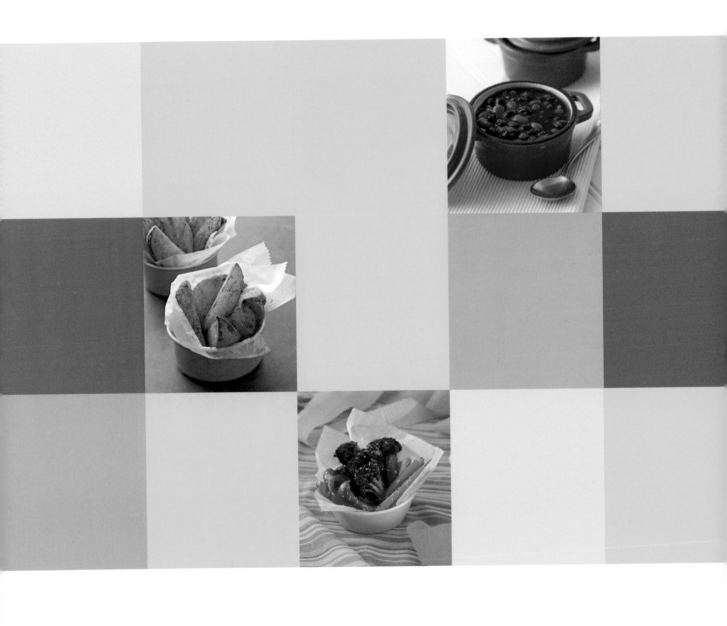

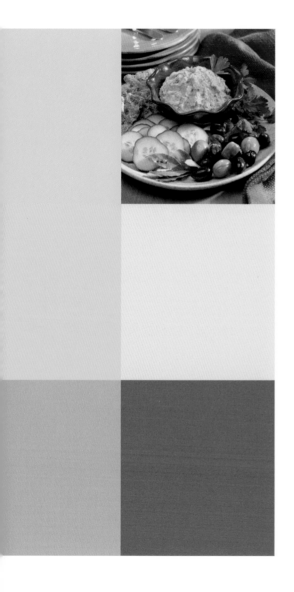

SOUP, SALAD, and SIDES

When we think of kids' favorite foods, soups and salads do not usually come to mind, but in my family hearty soups, salads, and sides are some of my kids' favorite dishes. For a light meal, mix and match a side and soup or salad. Some of my favorite recipes are in this chapter. Enjoy.

Easy Zucchini Soup

This creamy soup is simple to make. I find that even kids who do not like zucchini enjoy this soup.

1 tablespoon (15 ml) olive oil

1 sweet onion, diced

1 pound (455 g) zucchini, washed and sliced

1 can (15 ounces or 425 g) white beans or cannellini beans, drained

4 cups (946 ml) chicken or vegetable broth

Dash of salt, pepper, and nutmeg

1. Heat the oil in a large saucepan and sauté the onion and zucchini until tender.
2. In a food processor, purée the beans until smooth. Add a little water or broth if needed to achieve a smooth consistency. Pour into a bowl and set aside.
3. Add the sautéed onion and zucchini into the food processor and process until smooth; add a little broth to achieve a smooth consistency.
4. Pour the vegetable mixture into the saucepan and cook over medium heat. Add the bean purée and the remaining broth. Heat thoroughly and season with salt, pepper, and nutmeg to taste.

Yield: 8 servings

Chinese Pork Soup

This Asian-flavored soup is one of my kids' favorites. If you do not like pork, try ground turkey.

  1 tablespoon (8 g) corn, tapioca, or arrowroot starch

  1 tablespoon (6 g) fresh minced ginger

  1 pound (455 g) lean ground pork

  1 teaspoon (2.8 g) garlic

  5 cups (1.2 L) chicken or vegetable broth

  1 tablespoon (15 ml) gluten-free tamari

  2 cups (280 g) gluten-free vermicelli or spaghetti noodles, cooked and chopped

  1 cup (70 g) mushrooms, sliced

  ¼ cup (25 g) scallions, thinly sliced

  2 teaspoons (10 ml) olive oil

  1 cup (35 g) chopped bok choy or watercress

  Salt and pepper

1. In a large bowl mix together the starch, ginger, pork, and garlic. Form into 20 two-inch (5-cm) balls; set aside.

2. In a large pot bring the broth and tamari to a boil. Add the noodles and mushrooms. Gently drop in the meat balls and bring to a boil. Reduce heat and simmer for 12 minutes.

3. Stir in the bok choy or watercress . Remove from heat. Stir in the oil and scallions.

Yield: 6 servings

Salsa Soup

This is a pleasing soup that can be made with or without chicken.

1 tablespoon (15 ml) olive oil

1 tablespoon (8 g) millet or corn flour (optional)

½ cup (65 g) chopped onion

½ cup (60 g) chopped green bell pepper

4 cups (950 ml) water

2 chicken or vegetable bouillon cubes

1¾ cups (455 g) chunky salsa

½ teaspoon (1.1 g) ground cumin

1 can (15 ounces or 420 g) black beans, drained

1 can (15 ounces or 420 g) kidney or pinto beans, drained

2 cups (280 g) cooked diced or shredded chicken

1 tablespoon (15 ml) vegetable oil, for frying

6 corn tortillas cut into ½-inch (1.3-cm) strips or tortilla chips (optional)

1. In a large pot, heat the olive oil and the flour until you have made a paste. Add the onions and bell peppers and cook for 1 minute. Add the water, bouillon cubes, salsa, cumin, beans, and chicken. Bring to a boil and then reduce heat to medium and let simmer. Cook, covered, for 10 minutes.

2. In a frying pan, heat the vegetable oil and fry the tortilla pieces until crunchy, about 1 minute on each side. Sprinkle tortilla "chips" in soup or over individual bowls.

Yield: 8 servings

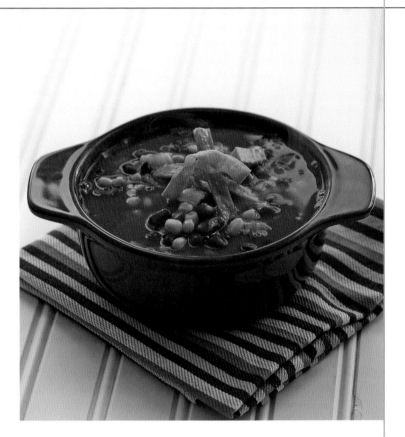

Outgrowing Food Allergies

Though it may prove difficult now to deal with your child's food allergies, take heart. Food allergies are frequently outgrown—especially milk, egg, and soybean allergies.

Harvest Soup

Both vegetables and fruit deliver nutrients, and the smooth and sweet flavors remind me of autumn. Omit the seasonings and this makes the perfect baby food!

    1 butternut squash

    3 cups (710 ml) vegetable broth

    1 large sweet potato or parsnip

    2 carrots

    2 green apples

    3 tablespoons (45 g) olive oil

    ½ teaspoon (1 g) fresh ginger, minced

    Salt and pepper

1. Peel and cube the butternut squash. Place squash and broth in a large stock pot. Bring to a boil and cook for 10 minutes. Lower heat to medium and chop and add the sweet potato, carrots, and apples. Cook until tender, about 10 more minutes.

2. With a slotted spoon, scoop out the vegetables while tilting the spoon to drain the liquid and place in a food processor or blender. Blend until all of the vegetables are smooth. Add a little broth if they're too thick.

3. Pour the purée back into the broth. Turn the heat up to medium-high. Add the ginger, stirring constantly until soup comes to a boil and then reduce heat to low. Add salt and pepper to taste.

4. For baby food: Cook vegetables and apples in water instead of broth and omit ginger, salt, and pepper. Let mixture cool in the refrigerator. Spoon into ice cube trays and wrap with foil. Freeze. To defrost, place 1 cube into a saucepan and bring to room temperature over low heat. Test temperature first before feeding to the baby.

Yield: 6 servings

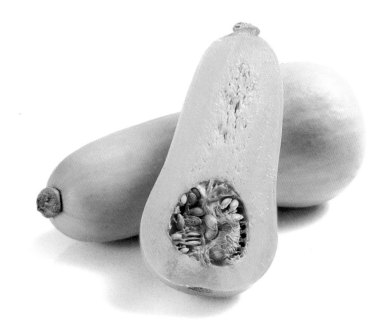

Chicken Noodle Soup

This simple soup is on everyone's favorite comfort food list. Some scientific evidence concludes that certain chicken soup recipes might actually help fight colds. Regardless, there is something about warm chicken noodle soup that seems to make you feel better when you're under the weather; but don't limit this quick soup to only when you or your kids are sick—it's great anytime. Add more vegetables for extra nutrients if desired.

2 teaspoons (10 ml) olive oil

1 cup (140 g) cooked, cubed chicken

½ white onion, chopped

3 carrots, scrubbed and sliced

2 celery stalks, chopped

¼ teaspoon (0.4 g) poultry seasoning

5 cups (1.2 liters) water

3 chicken bouillon cubes

1 cup (140 g) cooked rice spaghetti, chilled

Salt and pepper

1. In a medium pot, combine oil, chicken, onion, carrots, and celery. Cook for 2 minutes on medium-high heat. Add the poultry seasoning.

2. Add the water and bouillon cubes; stir until dissolved. Cook uncovered for 15 minutes over medium heat.

3. Chop the spaghetti into 2-inch (5-cm) pieces. Add to soup and stir for 3 minutes. Add salt and pepper to taste. Serve.

Yield: 8 servings

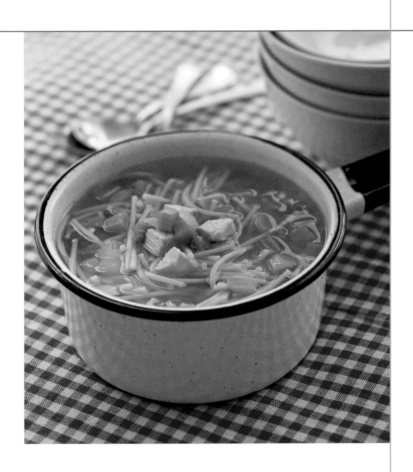

SOUP, SALADS, AND SIDES **157**

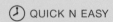

Teriyaki Veggie Spears

Treating Allergic Reactions

Although anaphylaxis requires immediate attention and a call to 911, most symptoms associated with an allergy can be eased right away with an anti-allergy medication that contains diphenhydramine. These antihistamines block the chemicals that cause allergic symptoms. Check with your doctor about which medication to have on hand if you have a child with a food allergy.

Steamed or baked vegetables can be downright bland. By glazing them with this great teriyaki sauce, the flave-o-meter goes way up, and little ones eat all their vegetables. Thank you, Lori, for this great idea!

> 1 pound (455 g) fresh vegetables (asparagus, carrots, broccoli, or mushrooms)
>
> ⅓ cup (80 ml) gluten-free tamari
>
> 1 tablespoon (15 ml) olive or vegetable oil
>
> ¼ cup (85 g) honey
>
> ¼ cup (30 g) white flax seeds

1. Preheat oven to 425°F (220°C, or gas mark 7).
2. Clean and cut the vegetables into long spears. Spray a broiling pan with vegetable oil spray and arrange the vegetables in the pan. Mix the tamari, oil, and honey. Drizzle over the veggies. Sprinkle with the flax seeds. Bake for about 10 minutes. Let cool before serving. They are tasty cold, too!

Yield: 2 cups (300 g)

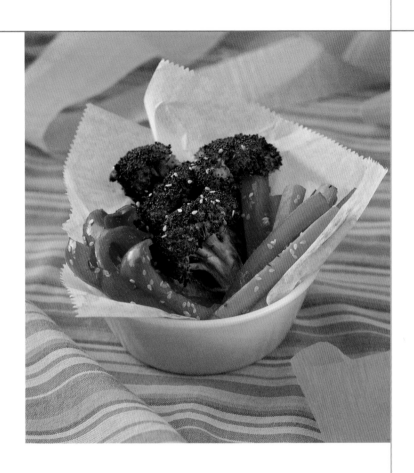

Curried Rice

Gluten-Free Resources
Thankfully, more and more places recognize the need for gluten-free products. Check out these companies that specialize in gluten-free products:

Cecilia's Gluten-Free Grocery
(800) 491-2760
www.glutenfreegrocery
.com

Gluten Solutions
(888) 845-8836
www.glutensolutions.com

Gluten-Free Mall
(online only)
www.glutenfreemall.com

My children do not usually enjoy spicy things, but they do like this mildly spicy, sweet rice dish. Add a fruit salad and some baked fish or chicken on the side to make a nice meal. This sweet rice is a great way to give kids wholesome grains.

1 tablespoon (15 ml) olive oil

¼ cup (35 g) chopped white onion

½ cup (60 g) chopped celery

1 cup (130 g) chopped carrots

⅔ cup (110 g) long-grain white rice

1 vegetable bouillon cube

1¼ cups (300 ml) water

1 teaspoon (2 g) curry powder

⅓ cup (50 g) currants

¼ cup (15 g) chopped fresh parsley

¼ cup (30 g) chopped roasted sunflower seeds

1. Heat oil in a large skillet and add the onion, celery, and carrots. Add the rice and cook for 1 minute or until rice starts to change color. Dissolve the bouillon cube in the water and pour into skillet. Add the curry powder and the currants; cover and cook over medium-low heat for 25 to 30 minutes or until rice is tender. Stir in the parsley and the sunflower seeds.

Yield: 4 servings

Taco Salad

Double this recipe for a large crowd. You will be surprised at how filling this salad is. This is a great hearty meal that delivers protein and fiber.

½ pound (225 g) ground beef

1 teaspoon (2.8 g) garlic powder

1 teaspoon (3 g) onion salt

1 tablespoon (7.5 g) chili powder

1 head romaine lettuce

1 can (15 ounces or 420 g) kidney beans, drained

1 can (15 ounces or 420 g) black beans, drained

½ cup (60 g) shredded jicama

1 medium cucumber, sliced

¼ cup (15 g) chopped cilantro

¼ cup (25 g) sliced scallions

1 avocado, sliced

1 firm tomato, chopped

1 cup (115 g) crushed tortilla chips (optional)

1 recipe Ranch Dressing or Salsa Vinaigrette (page 144)

1. In a skillet, brown the beef over medium heat. Add the garlic powder, onion salt, and chili powder. Cook until beef is no longer pink. Drain fat; set aside to cool.

2. Clean and chop the lettuce and place in a large bowl. Add the beans, jicama, cucumber, cilantro, scallions, avocado, and tomato. Sprinkle with meat and tortilla chips. Serve with desired dressing on the side or over the top.

Yield: 8 servings

Tortilla Chips Alternative
Can't have tortilla chips? The next time you bake the Quick Savory Crackers (page 42) reserve some for a crunchy topping for your soups and salads.

Mediterranean Veggies

Variation:
You can use purchased dressing instead of the vinegar and oil, if desired.

Try roasting the mixed vegetables instead of boiling them. It's a different twist to this delicious side dish.

> 5 cups (650 g) combination of your choice carrots, butternut squash, parsnips, zucchini, and broccoli, cooked, cooled, peeled, and cubed
>
> ½ red bell pepper, thinly sliced
>
> ½ red onion, thinly sliced
>
> ⅓ cup (80 ml) rice or red wine vinegar
>
> ¼ cup (60 ml) olive or canola oil
>
> ⅓ cup (20 g) fresh chopped oregano or parsley
>
> Salt and pepper to taste
>
> 2 tablespoons (5.3 g) chopped fresh or (9 g) dried basil
>
> 2 tablespoons (17 g) chopped olives (optional)

1. Combine all ingredients in a bowl. Cover and refrigerate for at least 30 minutes.

Yield: 6 to 8 servings

Mock Mayonnaise

This may seem to have odd ingredients in it, but it truly tastes really good. Currently, there are no egg-free, soy-free mayos on the market. This gives a creamy taste to salads, a great base for your dressings, and even acts as a nice dip for your veggies! Try different pepper mixes, like dill or Italian-seasoned. This mayo adds protein to your dishes and is low in fat!

1 can (15 ounces or 430 g) white navy or cannellini beans, drained, not rinsed

¼ cup (60 ml) olive oil

2 teaspoons (5.3 g) corn, tapioca, or arrowroot starch

Dash of rice vinegar

Squeeze of lemon

Salt and pepper to taste

1. In a food processor, purée all ingredients until smooth. Add lemon juice and vinegar until you have reached the desired mayonnaise consistency.

Yield: 1½ cups (340 g)

The Food Allergen Labeling and Consumer Protection Act (FALCPA)
A food labeling law now requires food manufacturers to disclose in plain language whether products contain any of the top eight food allergens. FALCPA mandates that foods containing milk, eggs, fish, crustacean shellfish, peanuts, tree nuts, wheat, and soy must declare the food in plain language on the ingredient list or via the word "contains" followed by the name of the major food allergen or a parenthetical statement in the list of ingredients (e.g., albumin [egg]). Such ingredients must be listed even if they are present in colors, flavors, or spice blends. Additionally, manufacturers must list the specific nut or seafood that is used (e.g., almond, walnut, cashew; or tuna, salmon, shrimp, or lobster).

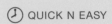

Bean Dip

For picky eaters who do not like meat, beans are a good source of protein and fiber. My family's favorite bean to use in this dip is chickpeas (also called garbanzo beans)—making this dip much like Middle Eastern hummus. Calling this bean dip instead of hummus may make it more appealing to some young children.

1 can (15 ounces or 420 g) beans (chickpea/garbanzo, black, navy, or pinto), undrained

1 tablespoon (15 ml) lemon juice

2 teaspoons (5.6 g) minced garlic

¼ teaspoon (1.5 g) salt

½ teaspoon ground (0.9 g) cayenne pepper

1 tablespoon (4 g) chopped cilantro

2 tablespoons (30 ml) olive oil or vegetable oil

Vegetables of your choice for dipping

Chips for dipping

1. In a food processor, blend beans, lemon juice, garlic, salt, cayenne pepper, cilantro, and oil until smooth. Add more oil if you prefer a thinner, smoother dip or drain the beans if you like a thicker paste. Cover and keep refrigerated. Use within the day.

2. Cut the vegetables into long spears. Place a bowl of dip in the center of a plate and arrange vegetables and chips around the bowl to serve.

Yield: about 2 cups (500 g) dip

Fiber Benefits

"Water-soluble fiber prevalent in oat bran, oatmeal, citrus fruit, and most types of beans seems to help clean out cholesterol. Round, irregularly shaped, buff-colored legumes, chickpeas are also called garbanzo beans or ceci. When you accompany chickpeas with vitamin C-rich foods like green peppers, the body makes better use of their nonheme iron." Serving fiber-rich foods to your kids from a young age will set them up for good eating habits as they get older. (Source: *Prevention* magazine's *Nutrition Advisor*, p. 35)

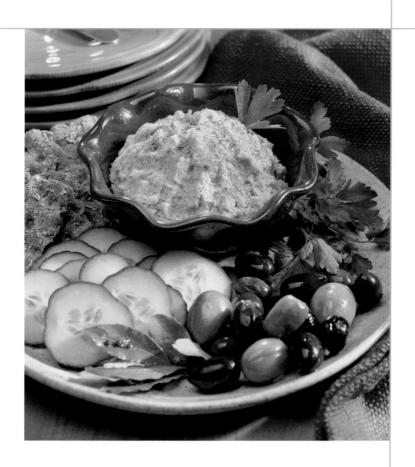

Spinach Dip

Spotlight on Jicama

Jicama (pronounced "hee-ca-ma") is a tropical legume that produces an edible fleshy taproot. It is native to Mexico and northern Central America and is widely cultivated there and in Southeast Asia. Jicama is most commonly eaten fresh. After the fibrous brown outer tissue of the root is peeled away, the crisp white flesh can be sliced, diced, or cut into strips for use as a garnish, in salads, or with dips. It is frequently served as a snack, sprinkled with lime or lemon juice and a dash of chili powder. Jicama remains crisp after boiling and serves as a textural substitute for water chestnuts. Jicama is similar in food value to white potatoes but with slightly fewer calories. Kids love its crunchy texture, and it makes a great dipper for these fun dip recipes.

Treat your children to a snack worthy of Popeye and packing a punch of vitamin A. By choosing carrots for dipping instead of crackers or bread, you'll give your little ones a beta-carotene wallop, too. What a yummy way to get in several servings of veggies a day!

- 1 cup (235 g) Mock Mayonnaise (see recipe page 163)
- 1 teaspoon (5 ml) gluten-free tamari
- ¼ cup (30 g) finely chopped red bell peppers
- ¼ cup (15 g) fresh, finely chopped parsley
- ¼ cup (25 g) chopped scallions
- ½ cup (65 g) chopped white onion
- ¼ cup (30 g) finely chopped jicama (optional)
- 1 package (8 ounces or 225 g) frozen chopped spinach, thawed and drained
- 1 teaspoon (2.1 g) ground black pepper
- ¼ teaspoon (0.5 g) ground cayenne pepper

1. In a large bowl, mix mock mayonnaise, tamari, bell pepper, parsley, scallions, onion, and jicama.
2. Stir in spinach, black pepper, and cayenne pepper. Refrigerate for 30 minutes and serve.

Yield: about 3 cups (700 g)

Mexican Layer "Creamy" Dip

Serve this favorite with chips or heated corn tortillas. Though mainly served as a snack, we sometimes make a meal out of this hearty dip. One-fifth of a medium avocado (1 ounce) has 50 calories and contributes nearly 20 vitamins and minerals, making it a healthy choice. Although high in fat, it delivers the healthy fats that your kids' hearts need for proper development.

- 1 can (16 ounces or 455 g) refried pinto or black beans
- 1 cup (225 g) canned cannellini or Great Northern beans, drained
- 2 teaspoons (5.2 g) chili powder
- 1 tablespoon (15 ml) olive or vegetable oil
- 1 cup (250 g) guacamole (see Sneaky Guacamole recipe, page 66)
- 1 cup (260 g) salsa or diced fresh tomatoes

1. Spread the refried beans on the bottom of an 8 × 8-inch (20 × 20-cm) baking dish.

2. In a food processor, purée the cannellini beans, chili powder, and oil. Layer this mixture over the refried beans. Spread the guacamole over and then top with the salsa or tomatoes. Serve immediately or cover and refrigerate for up to 24 hours.

Yeild: about 4½ cups

**Spotlight on
Cannellini Beans**
Cannellini bean = white kidney bean = fazolia bean You've probably already encountered this Italian bean in minestrone soup or a bean salad. It's prized for its smooth texture and nutty flavor, which kids seem to like. You can substitute fresh cannellini beans, Great Northern beans, navy beans, calypso beans, or flageolets. (Source: Cook's thesaurus at www. foodsubs.com)

Mexican-Style Baked Beans

Low-sugar variation:
Omit brown sugar
and molasses. Use 1
cup (240 g) sugar-free
ketchup in place of
regular ketchup.

Just a little variation on the old American favorite!

1 teaspoon (5 ml) vegetable oil

½ cup (65 g) chopped onions

¼ cup (60 g) brown sugar

one 15-ounce (420-g) can Mexican-seasoned pinquito beans

one 15-ounce (420-g) can pinto, black, or navy beans, drained

1 cup (250 g) barbecue sauce

½ cup (120 g) ketchup

3 tablespoons (45 ml) molasses

¼ cup (15 g) cilantro

Salt and pepper

1. In a pot combine oil, onions, and brown sugar. Cook for 1 minute. Add the beans, barbecue sauce, ketchup, and molasses. Cook on medium heat until mixture begins to boil. Turn heat to low, add the cilantro. Stir in the salt and pepper to taste. Cook on low for 30 minutes, covered. Let sit 10 minutes before serving.

Yield: 8 servings

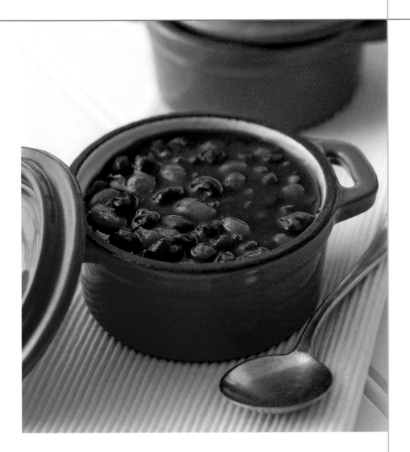

Celiac Diagnosis

It takes an average of ten years and just as many different physicians to be diagnosed with celiac disease, according to *Prevention* magazine's November 1, 2000, issue (Vol. 52, No. 11). If you suspect you or your child has celiac disease or another food allergy, ask your doctor about getting tested. And if you or your child has been suffering with celiac disease for a long time and only recently realized what the problem was, take heart. If you swear off gluten, most of the symptoms and problems associated with celiac disease disappear within six months.

Green Bean Bake

**Milk Allergies
More Common than
Previously Thought**
Before 1950, an allergy
to cow's milk was consid-
ered very rare, according
to the January 15, 2003,
edition of *The Indepen-
dent* (London, England).
But now, a French
research team has found
evidence to suspect that
milk allergies affect up
to 10 percent of infants
and 5 percent of older
children.

This is a family-pleasing side dish and complements any main
course. Making this from scratch lowers the sodium and adds
amazing flavor.

½ cup (60 g) white rice flour

½ teaspoon (1.5 g) garlic salt

½ teaspoon (1 g) pepper

2 tablespoons (30 ml) oil

½ white onion, sliced

1 cup (230 g) puréed white navy beans

½ cup (120 ml) alternative milk beverage

2 tablespoons (30 ml) gluten-free tamari

4 cups (500 g) fresh or frozen green beans, cut

1 cup (70 g) sliced mushrooms

1. Preheat oven to 350°F (180°C, or gas mark 4).

2. In a bowl, combine the flour, garlic salt, and pepper. Heat the
   oil in a skillet until hot. Toss the onion slices in the flour mixture
   and place in the hot skillet. Fry for 2 minutes or until golden.
   Set aside.

3. In a large bowl, mix the puréed beans, milk alternative, and tamari.
   Stir in the green beans and mushrooms. Pour into a 9-inch
   (22.5-cm) baking pan. Top with onions. Bake for 30 minutes.

Yield: 6 servings

Fried Rice

Have a theme dinner night: Include this side dish with Teriyaki Veggie Spears (recipe page 158), and use the same sauce for cooked chicken strips. This home-cooked version of fried rice gives you restaurant-quality flavors but is much healthier for you.

2 tablespoons (30 ml) olive or vegetable oil

1 teaspoon (1.8 g) ground ginger

2 carrots, scrubbed and sliced

½ cup (55 g) cubed cooked ham (optional)

3 cups (500 g) brown or white rice, cooked

¼ cup (25 g) sliced scallions

2 tablespoons (30 ml) gluten-free tamari

1 cup (130 g) frozen peas

1. In a large skillet, combine oil, ginger, carrots, and ham. Cook for 1 minute. Add the rice, scallions, tamari, and peas. Stir. Cover and let cook for 6 minutes. Stir in additional tamari, if desired.

Yield: 5 servings

Red Potatoes

These are my favorite seasoned potatoes and are especially good with Happy Burgers. Baking your potatoes is always a healthier choice than frying.

8 red potatoes, scrubbed and cut into wedges

3 tablespoons (45 ml) olive oil

1½ teaspoons (3 g) pepper

¼ teaspoon (1.5 g) salt

½ teaspoon (1.4 g) garlic powder

2 tablespoons (14 g) paprika

1 teaspoon (2.6 g) chili powder

1. Preheat oven to 400°F (200°C, or gas mark 6).
2. In a large pot bring 8 cups (1.9 liters) of salted water to a boil. Place the potatoes in the pot and boil for 2 minutes, or until barely soft (you want them to be firm, not mushy). Strain and place in a large bowl; toss with oil.
3. Add remaining ingredients and stir to coat.
4. Place on a greased baking sheet and bake for 20 minutes or until golden and crisp. Serve.

Yield: 8 servings

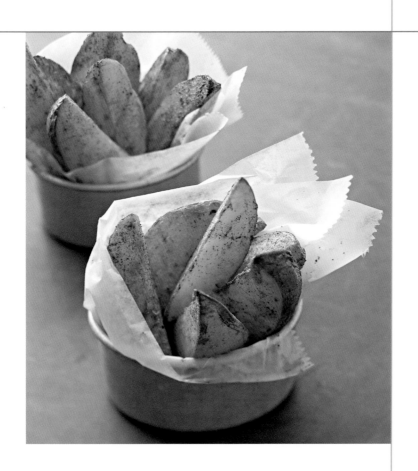

Mixed Veggie Hash

Variation:
For pancakes, form
patties and fry a few
at a time, 5 minutes
on each side.

Rely on Olive Oil

Olive oil is perfect for today's healthy lifestyle because it has no cholesterol and is one of the oils highest in monounsaturated fats. For people who must avoid hydrogenated oil, olive oil is a good choice for cooking, frying, and replacing butter and oil in baked goods. It ranges in flavors from mild to strongly fruity; have your kids do a taste test to see which they like best.

Try this in place of potato hash browns for more nutrients and lower fat.

2 cups (250 g) grated mixed vegetables, such as zucchini, parsnip, carrots, and yellow squash

¼ cup (35 g) grated onion

2 tablespoons (8 g) chopped cilantro (optional)

¼ cup (28 g) flax meal

½ teaspoon (3 g) salt

2 teaspoons (10 ml) olive oil

1. In a large bowl, combine all ingredients.
2. Grease a large skillet and heat over medium-high heat. Spread vegetable mixture evenly across the bottom of the pan. Cover and cook for 10 minutes. With a spatula, flip sections over and cook an additional 5 minutes.

Yield: 5 servings

Mock Top Ramen Soup

This noodle recipe mimics the most popular, packaged ramen noodle meals on the market—without the possible allergens.

    2 teaspoons (10 ml) olive oil

    2 carrots, scrubbed and diced small

    ¼ teaspoon (0.5 g) ground ginger

    1 cup (110 g) diced cooked ham or chicken (optional)

    5 cups (1.2 liters) beef, chicken, or vegetable broth

    2 tablespoons (30 ml) gluten-free tamari

    ¼ cup (25 g) scallions, chopped

    1 cup (130 g) frozen peas

    8 ounces (225 g) gluten-free thin Asian noodles or spaghetti

1. In a medium pot, combine oil, carrots, ginger, and ham. Cook for 1 minute. Add the broth, tamari, scallions, and peas.

2. In a separate pot, bring 2 cups (475 ml) of water to a boil and add the Asian noodles. Let sit 2 minutes or until soft. If using spaghetti noodles, cook according to directions. Rinse with cold water and chop into 8-inch (20-cm) pieces. Add to soup, stir, and serve.

Yield: 5 servings

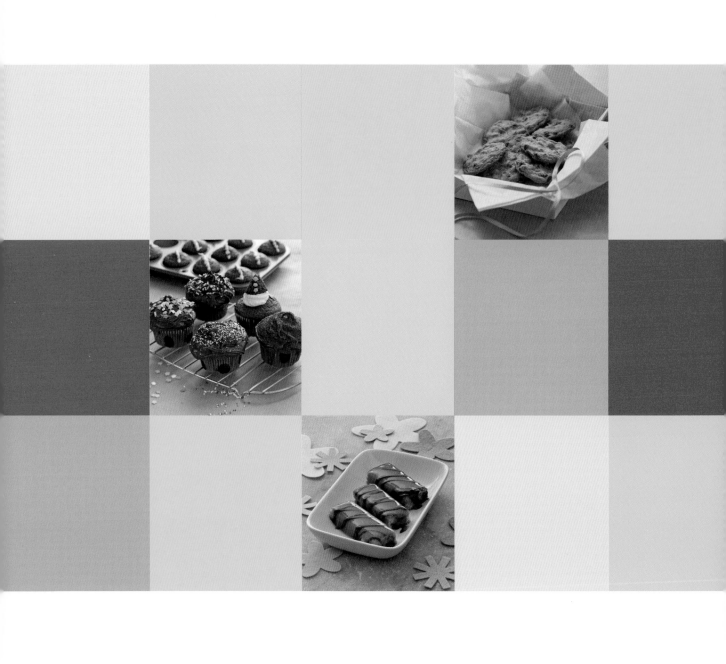

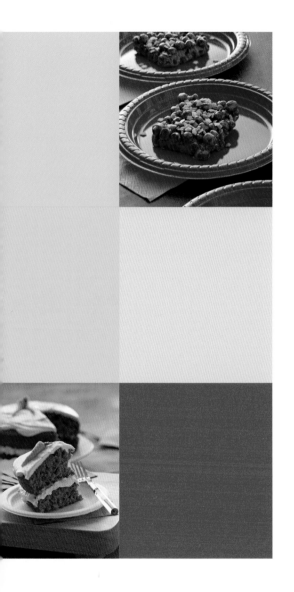

SWEETS and TREATS

Gooey desserts, tasty candies, and yummy creations—every kid loves sweets! And every child deserves a little taste-bud fun occasionally. This section caters to a child's sweet tooth. So many parents with little ones suffering from food allergies can't find yummy treats that won't make their children sick. These recipes will put a smile (and an icing smear!) on any child's face and won't make a wee one with food allergies ill. So go ahead, pass out the cookies, cakes, and pies.

Vanilla Chip Cookies

Going Gluten-Free? Don't Get Discouraged!

When a parent discovers that a child has an allergy to wheat, suddenly it seems like every food is off limits—so many of our packaged foods and snacks do include flour as a key ingredient. But many snack foods, like the ones in this chapter, contain no gluten whatsoever. Part of feeding your child begins with taking a deep breath and recognizing all the allergy-free things we *can* eat!

Nobody ever believes that this awesome cookie is made with only rice flour! Use your choice of flavored, allergy-safe chips.

½ cup (100 g) vegetable shortening

½ cup (115 g) dark or light brown sugar

½ cup (100 g) white sugar

2 teaspoons (10 ml) vanilla extract

3 cups (375 g) white or brown rice flour

½ cup (60 g) tapioca flour

2 teaspoons (5.4 g) corn, tapioca, or arrowroot starch

½ teaspoon salt

1 teaspoon baking powder

3 to 4 teaspoons water

2 cups (350 g) allergy-safe semisweet chocolate

1. In a mixer, combine the shortening and sugars. Scrape down the sides of the bowl and add the vanilla. Mix again for about 10 seconds.

2. Add in rice flour, tapioca flour, starch, salt, baking powder, and water. Blend on medium speed until dough is combined. Remove bowl from mixer and stir in chocolate chips.

3. Firmly pack cookie dough in a 1- to 2-inch (2.5- to 5-cm) cookie dough scoop and place cookies next to each other on a lined baking sheet. (You may need two baking sheets.) Place the baking sheet(s) in the freezer and freeze for 30 minutes. To store, remove dough from baking sheet, place in a resealable plastic freezer bag, and refreeze for up to 2 months.

4. To bake, preheat oven to 350°F (180°C, or gas mark 4). Take out desired number of cookies and place on a baking sheet. Bring cookies to room temperature, about 15 minutes. You may also thaw them in the refrigerator. Bake for 8 minutes. Leave on baking sheet until cooled completely. Remove to a cooling rack and let sit for about 1 hour. Cookies should be able to hold their shape. Store in a covered container.

Yield: about 3 dozen cookies

Quick and Easy
Chocolate Chip Cookies

These cookies are so quick and about as easy to make as buying the refrigerated cookie dough from the store but without the unhealthy, unpronounceable ingredients!

⅓ cup (80 ml) vegetable oil

1 cup (225 g) packed brown sugar

2 teaspoons (10 ml) vanilla extract

¼ teaspoon (1.5 ml) salt

1 cup (125 g) white rice flour

½ cup (60 g) tapioca flour

1 tablespoon (8 g) corn, tapioca, or arrowroot starch

1 teaspoon (4.6 g) baking powder

¼ cup (60 ml) plus 2 tablespoons (90 ml) water

1 cup (175 g) allergy-safe semisweet chocolate chips

1. Preheat oven to 350°F (180°C, or gas mark 4).

2. In a mixer or by hand, stir together oil, brown sugar, vanilla, and salt. Add the flours, starch, and baking powder and mix on low speed. While mixing, slowly pour in the water until the dough is smooth. Stir in the chocolate chips.

3. Use a small ice cream/cookie scoop or drop dough by table-spoon onto a baking sheet, spacing the cookies about 2 inches (5 cm) apart (about 6 cookies per baking sheet).

4. Bake for 12 to 15 minutes or until golden around the edges and soft in the center. For softer cookies, remove from oven before they get too golden—around 12 minutes. Let cool on baking sheet for less than 1 minute. Remove with a flat spatula and place on a flat surface to cool completely.

Yield: about 2 dozen cookies

Chewy Chocolate Chip Cookies

Miss the chewy chocolaty chip cookies that grandma would make? Here you go! These have recently become my family's favorite cookie.

1 cup (225 g) brown sugar

¼ cup (60 ml) vegetable oil

½ cup (100 g) vegetable shortening

2 teaspoons (10 ml) vanilla extract

1 cup plus 2 tablespoons (140 g) white rice flour

½ teaspoon (2.3 g) baking soda

¼ teaspoon (1.5 g) salt

2 cups (350 g) allergy-safe chocolate chips

1. Preheat oven to 350°F (180°C, or gas mark 4).
2. Using a mixer, beat together the brown sugar, oil, shortening, and vanilla. Add the flour, baking soda, and salt. Mix until smooth. Stir in chocolate chips.
3. Using a small cookie dough scoop, drop dough onto baking sheet about 2 inches (5 cm) apart.
4. Bake for 8 to 10 minutes, depending on size of cookie. These cookies get golden quickly. Remove from oven when the centers are a little soft. Let cookies cool completely on baking sheet. Remove with a spatula.

Yield: 24 cookies

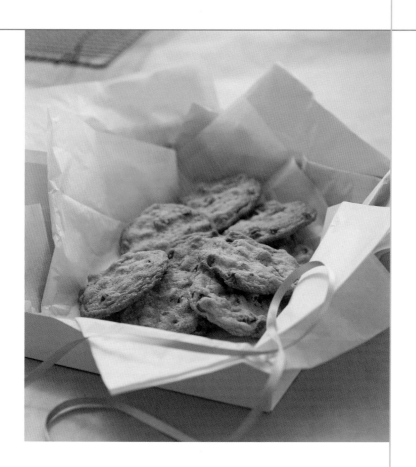

Gourmet Oatmeal Chocolate Chunk Cookies

These cookies are worthy of selling at a café!

½ cup (100 g) sugar

½ cup (115 g) brown sugar

1 tablespoon (15 ml) alternative milk beverage or water

1 cup (200 g) vegetable shortening

1 tablespoon (15 ml) vanilla extract

1⅔ cup (208 g) white or brown rice flour

1⅓ cup (107 g) old-fashioned certified gluten-free oats

1 teaspoon (4.6 g) baking soda

1 teaspoon (4.6 g) baking powder

½ teaspoon (3 g) salt

one 3.5-ounce (100 g) chocolate bar, chopped into small chunks

1. Preheat oven to 350°F (180°C, or gas mark 4).

2. In a mixer, cream together sugars, milk alternative, shortening, and vanilla. Mix in remaining ingredients except the chocolate. Gently fold in the chocolate chunks.

3. Using a small or medium-size cookie dough scoop, drop dough on a greased baking sheet, allowing room for spreading. Slightly flatten the tops of the cookies.

4. Bake for 8 to 10 minutes; cookies should be soft in the middle. Do not overbake. Cool cookies completely on baking sheet and then remove with a spatula.

Yield: 36 cookies

Excellent Sunflower Shortbread Cookies

This is like a "nutty" shortbread. Although it's in a cookie, the sunflower butter gives your kids a great source of protein.

½ cup (100 g) vegetable shortening

1 cup (225 g) brown sugar

1 teaspoon (5 ml) vanilla extract

½ cup (130 g) sunflower butter

½ cup (60 g) white or brown rice flour

½ cup (60 g) tapioca flour

1 tablespoon (8 g) corn, tapioca, or arrowroot starch

½ teaspoon (3 g) salt

1 teaspoon (4.6 g) baking powder

1. Preheat oven to 350°F (180°C, or gas mark 4).
3. In a mixer, cream together the shortening, brown sugar, vanilla, and sunflower butter. Mix in the remaining ingredients.
4. With a large cookie dough scoop, drop dough onto a baking sheet about 3 inches (7.5 cm) apart. Bake for 15 to 20 minutes or until golden. Let cool on baking sheet completely and remove with a spatula.

Yield: 24 cookies

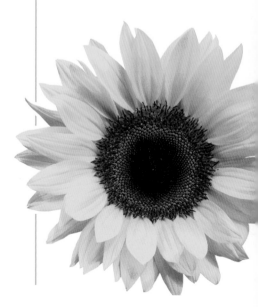

Sugar Cookies

Sugar Cookies—a Universal Treat!

Virtually every culture has its version of sugar cookies. Arab countries decorate the cookies with a pistachio or almond in the center of each, Greeks put a clove as a decoration, and many cultures heavily dust the top with powdered sugar. No matter where you're from or how you decorate them, sugar cookies are a favorite. Now with my allergy-friendly version, every child can have a sugar cookie!

This is an old-fashioned favorite that my family loves. If you keep the dough well chilled and really work with it, these rolled-out cookies are delicate and delicious.

½ cup (125 g) unsweetened applesauce

1 cup (200 g) sugar

2 teaspoons (10 ml) vanilla extract

½ cup (100 g) vegetable shortening

¼ teaspoon (1.5 g) salt

½ teaspoon (2.3 g) baking soda

½ teaspoon (1.5 g) cream of tartar

1½ cups (185 g) white rice flour

1 cup (125 g) tapioca flour

1. Preheat oven to 350°F (180°C, or gas mark 4).

2. In a mixer, cream together applesauce, sugar, vanilla, shortening, and salt. Add the remaining ingredients and mix at low speed, increasing to medium speed until batter is smooth.

3. Pinch off 1 to 2 teaspoons of dough and roll into balls. Place on a baking sheet and flatten slightly. Or to make decorated cookie shapes with cookie cutters, divide dough into fourths. Place one section of dough between two pieces of nonstick parchment paper. With a rolling pin, roll dough into a flat ½-inch (1.2-cm) disk. Use a cookie cutter to cut out shapes and then with a flat spatula gently remove the cookie shapes to a greased baking sheet. Collect remaining scrap dough and repeat process.

4. Bake for 12 to 15 minutes or until the cookies are darker around the edges and firm in the centers. Watch the cookies to make sure they don't get too golden. Remove from baking sheet with a flat spatula and place on a flat surface to cool.

Yield: 36 cookies

Brown Sugar Dough

This dough is perfect for sweet tarts, pastries, and bar cookie bases.

½ cup (100 g) vegetable shortening

2 cups (250 g) rice flour

1¼ cups (285 g) brown sugar, packed

½ teaspoon (2.5 ml) vanilla extract

½ cup (65 g) corn, tapioca, or arrowroot starch

¼ teaspoon (1.5 g) salt

3 tablespoons (45 ml) alternative milk beverage or water

1. In a food processor, combine all ingredients. Pulse until the mixture resembles cornmeal.
2. Remove dough from processor and divide in half. Wrap each half in waxed paper and chill until ready to use.

Yield: about 3 cups (675 g)

A Peanut Vaccine?

Peanut allergies afflict 1.5 million Americans and kill about 100 people a year. The *Globe* newspaper reported in October 2002 that scientists are "closing in on treatments for the most deadly of all food allergies"—peanuts—with a possible vaccine. The FDA approved "fast-track" testing for the first-ever drug to weaken allergic reactions to peanuts. One of the doctors working on the vaccine, Dr. Wesley Burks of Duke University, hopes that it will "lessen the chances significantly that an accidental ingestion would be life-threatening." Using a similar method, immunotherapy helped children with egg allergies tame their allergic reactions, say Dr. Burks and Dr. Stacie Jones at Arkansas Children's Hospital in a small study published in *The Journal of Allergy and Clinical Immunology* in January 2009.

Fun Cut-Outs

More Cookie Fun

For cookies on sticks that are fun to decorate, prepare dough according to directions. Use an ice cream scoop to gather a ball of dough, place onto waxed paper sprayed with cooking oil, and flatten slightly. Insert stick halfway in. Bake for about 10 minutes. Cool completely before removing from pan. Large craft stores have a great baking section where you can find decorative candies, scoops, and cookie pop sticks—and cellophane bags to package them in for gift-giving!

These taste great and are perfect for school parties.

¼ cup (60 ml) orange juice or lemonade concentrate

¼ cup (60 ml) water

½ cup (50 g) powdered sugar (contains corn starch, use corn-free recipe on page 82)

½ cup (100 g) superfine sugar

2 teaspoons (10ml) vanilla extract

½ cup (100 g) vegetable shortening

¼ teaspoon (1.5 g) salt

1 teaspoon (1.7 g) orange zest

½ teaspoon (2.3 g) baking soda

½ teaspoon cream of tartar

1½ cups (185 g) white rice flour

1 cup (125 g) tapioca flour

1. Preheat oven to 350°F (180°C, or gas mark 4).

2. In a mixer, cream together orange juice, water, sugars, vanilla, shortening, salt, and zest. Add the remaining cookie ingredients and mix on low, gradually increasing to medium speed until the batter is smooth.

3. Pinch off 1 to 2 teaspoons of dough and roll into balls. Place on a baking sheet. Flatten slightly.

4. Bake for about 12 to 15 minutes. Remove from baking sheet with a spatula and place on a flat surface to cool.

Yield: about 36 cookies

Fruit Bars

For Cookie Base:

½ cup (115 g) packed brown sugar

½ cup (60 g) tapioca flour

1 cup (125 g) white or brown rice flour

½ teaspoon (1.2 g) ground cinnamon

½ teaspoon (2.3 g) baking powder

Dash of salt

¼ cup (60 ml) vegetable oil

¼ cup (60 ml) water

For Strudel Topping:

¼ cup (60 ml) vegetable oil

1 cup (225 g) packed brown sugar

1 tablespoon (15 ml) water

½ cup (60 g) white or brown rice flour

1 cup (80 g) certified gluten-free rolled oats, rolled rice, quinoa, or buckwheat flakes

¼ cup (30 g) tapioca flour

1 teaspoon (2.3 g) cinnamon

For Filling:

1 jar (10.25 ounces or 287 g) your choice of allergy-safe jam or preserves

1. Preheat oven to 350°F (180°C, or gas mark 4).

2. To make the cookie base: Combine all cookie base ingredients in a food processor and process until dough is smooth. Press dough into a 9 × 13-inch (23 × 33-cm) pan. Wet your hands if dough is too sticky. Bake for 10 minutes; set aside to cool. Do not turn off oven.

3. To make the strudel topping: In a food processor (no need to clean it after making the cookie base), add topping ingredients and pulse mixture until it forms pea-sized pieces. Set aside.

4. Spread filling over cooled crust. Sprinkle strudel topping evenly over the preserves. Bake for 30 to 35 minutes or until golden on top. Cool for one hour or until room temperature. Cover and place in the refrigerator. When chilled, cut into bars.

Yield: about 24 bars

Caramel Layer Bars

This is a treat that I missed out on as a kid, but you do not have to!

For Bars:

1 recipe Brown Sugar Dough (page 185)

¼ cup (50 g) vegetable shortening

1 cup (225 g) dark brown sugar

1½ cups (150 g) powdered sugar (contains cornstarch, use corn-free recipe on page 103)

4 (20 ml) to 6 (30 ml) teaspoons alternative milk beverage

For Topping:

1½ cups (260 g) allergy-safe semisweet chocolate chips

2 teaspoons (8 g) vegetable shortening

1. Preheat oven to 375°F (190°C, or gas mark 5).

2. To make the bars: In a 9-inch (22.5-cm) square cake pan, press Brown Sugar Dough in evenly and prick with a fork. Bake for 20 minutes or until lightly golden. Remove and let cool in the pan.

3. Combine the shortening, brown sugar, powdered sugar, and 4 teaspoons of milk alternative in a small saucepan. Cook over low heat, constantly stirring with a whisk. If mixture is too thick, add remaining 2 teaspoons milk alternative. Stir until smooth. Pour mixture over the cookie bottom. Let cool.

4. To make the topping: In a microwave-safe bowl, melt the chocolate for 1 minute, stopping at 30 seconds to stir. Add shortening and stir until melted and smooth. Pour over cooled caramel mixture and spread evenly to the edges of the pan. Cool completely. Place in the refrigerator for 30 minutes or until chilled. Cut into squares with a sharp knife. Best kept refrigerated.

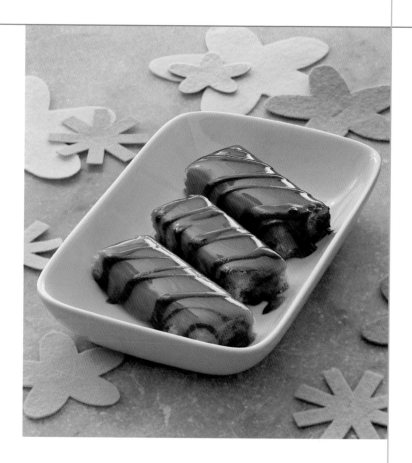

5. For candy look-alikes: Before adding the chocolate, cut cooled caramel-covered base into finger-sized bars. Place bars on a parchment-lined baking sheet and pour chocolate over each cookie until all are completely covered with chocolate. Put back into refrigerator to cool. Serve or wrap in parchment and freeze in a resealable plastic bag. They taste great frozen, too!

Yield: 12 bars

Caramel Wheels

Gluten-Free Caramel
Often gluten is found in caramel-flavored syrups. Make this caramel recipe and store it in a plastic container for up to 2 weeks. Use it to create homemade ice-cream sundaes or dip apple wedges!

1 recipe Brown Sugar Dough (page 185)

¼ cup (50 g) vegetable shortening

1 cup (225 g) brown sugar

2 cups (200 g) powdered sugar (contains cornstarch, use corn-free recipe on page 103)

4 teaspoons (20 ml) alternative milk beverage

1 cup (70 g) allergy-safe mini semisweet chocolate chips or flaked coconut (optional)

1. Preheat oven to 350°F (180°C, or gas mark 4).

2. Divide Brown Sugar Dough into two disks and put between two oil-sprayed pieces of waxed paper. Roll out to ⅛-inch (0.3 cm) thick. With a 2- or 3-inch (5- or 7.5-cm) round cookie cutter, cut out cookies. Gather scraps of dough and repeat process until all dough has been used. If cookies start sticking, spray with cooking oil. Place 1 inch (2.5 cm) apart on a greased baking sheet. Bake for about 10 minutes. Remove cookies to rack to cool.

3. Combine the shortening, brown sugar, powdered sugar, and 4 teaspoons of milk alternative in a small saucepan. Cook over low heat, stirring constantly with a whisk. Stir until smooth. Mixture will be thick.

4. Turn cookies bottom-side up and spread 1 tablespoon (15 ml) caramel on half of the cookies. Sandwich together with remaining cookies.

5. Fill a small bowl with mini chocolate chips or coconut. Squeeze the cookie slightly so it oozes out a little caramel and roll in the chocolate chips or coconut. Repeat with all cookies.

Yield: About 24 sandwiches

Honey Graham Crackers

These crackers are the perfect hearty cookie to take to school, on trips, or to munch on the go. They are also a good source of fiber.

½ cup (115 g) dark brown sugar

½ cup (100 g) vegetable shortening

½ cup (120 ml) honey

1 teaspoon (5 ml) vanilla extract

1½ cups (190 g) brown rice flour

½ cup (50 g) rice bran

1 cup (112 g) ground flaxseeds

1 teaspoon (4.6 g) baking powder

½ teaspoon (2.3 g) baking soda

½ teaspoon (3 g) salt

2 teaspoons (4.6 g) cinnamon

¼ cup (60 ml) milk

Extra rice flour for rolling

1. Preheat oven to 350°F (180°C, or gas mark 4).

2. In a mixer, cream together the sugar, shortening, honey, and vanilla until fluffy. Add the next 7 ingredients (through cinnamon). While mixing, slowly add in milk.

3. Divide the dough into 4 equal pieces. Roll each piece into a ball. If dough is sticky, refrigerate for 30 minutes or until firm.

4. Sprinkle some rice flour on a flat work surface. Cover 1 ball of dough with plastic wrap. With a rolling pin, roll out the dough into a 15 × 5-inch (37.5 × 13-cm) rectangle. With a knife, even out the edges into a perfect rectangle. To make these cookies look like packaged graham crackers, indent the rectangle in the center to look like two squares. Do not cut all the way through. Prick the surface with a fork. Repeat with remaining dough. Gently arrange rectangles on a greased baking sheet.

5. Bake crackers for 15 minutes or until lightly browned around the edges. Let cool on baking sheet. Remove to a flat surface.

Yield: About 24 cookies

Very Vanilla

Vanilla is one of the most popular flavorings in dessert making, and it's free of the 8 major allergens. It is derived from aromatic pods of a variety of orchid. The extract is made by dissolving the essential oil of the vanilla bean in an alcohol base. Use products labeled "pure" or "natural" vanilla ("imitation" or "essence" is not the same thing). Extract from Madagascar has the best quality. I use powdered vanilla and find it is very useful for sauces, custards, and a million-and-one sweet dishes or wherever a touch of vanilla flavor is required. I often double the amount of vanilla called for in all my recipes for added flavor.

Shortbread

Lower-Sugar Treats
You can use half the amount of sugar called for in my recipes and still get fabulous results. You can also substitute natural products for sugar, such as honey, fruit juice, juice concentrate, pure maple syrup, Whey Low, and rice syrup (look for one without barley). Natural food stores also carry all-natural sweeteners like Sucanat, stevia, xylitol, and lohan.

½ cup (100 g) vegetable shortening

1 cup (125 g) white rice flour

½ cup (65 g) corn, tapioca, or arrowroot starch

½ cup (50 g) powdered sugar (contains cornstarch, use corn-free recipe on page 103)

⅛ teaspoon (0.6 g) baking powder

⅛ teaspoon (.75 g) salt

1 teaspoon (5 ml) vanilla extract

1. Preheat oven to 350°F (180°C, or gas mark 4).

2. In a food processor, combine all ingredients and process for 1 minute. Once the dough comes together, remove from the food processor and use your hands to form the dough into a ball. Place on a greased baking sheet and shape into an even circle. Pinch the edges and use a sharp knife to cut into 8 slices. Do not separate the slices.

3. Bake for 17 minutes or until edges are golden but the centers are still white. Let sit for half an hour on baking sheet to cool. With a sharp knife, re-cut along the edges of each slice. Sprinkle with powdered sugar, if desired.

3. Here's a fun idea: Make your shortbread flavor of choice. When completely cooled, frost with frosting or pudding and top with fruits, candies, and fun sprinkles to make a yummy treat.

Yield: 8 slices

Tea Cakes

This is my favorite cookie. I think this is better than the wheat version.

- ½ cup (100 g) vegetable shortening
- ½ cup (100 g) sugar
- ¼ cup (60 ml) alternative milk beverage
- 1½ cups (185 g) white rice flour
- ½ cup (65 g) corn, tapioca, or arrowroot starch
- ½ teaspoon (2.3 g) baking powder
- 1 cup (100 g) powdered sugar (corn-free recipe on page 103)

1. Preheat oven to 350°F (180°C, or gas mark 4).
2. Mix the shortening and sugar. Mixture will look coagulated. Add the remaining cookie ingredients and blend until the dough is smooth.
3. Form dough into a ball, cover in plastic wrap, and refrigerate for 30 minutes. If dough becomes too firm, leave out at room temperature for a few minutes until dough is easier to work with.
4. Pinch off 1 to 2 teaspoons of dough and roll into a ball; repeat with remaining dough. Place on a baking sheet about 2 inches apart. Do not flatten.
5. Bake for 15 minutes or until cookies are golden around the bottom edges. Remove with a spatula and place on a flat surface to cool.
6. Sift powdered sugar heavily over each cookie

Yield: 40 cookies

For Lemon Tea Cakes:
After cookies cool, mix together 1 cup (100 g) powdered sugar and 3 tablespoons (45 ml) lemon juice concentrate. Spoon glaze over each cookie and cool until firm to the touch.

Lemon Berry Bars

My aunt loves lemon bars, and she totally approves of these! Berries add not only flavor, but also nutritional value.

For Crust:

½ cup (120 ml) fresh lemon juice

1 teaspoon (1.7 g) lemon zest

½ cup (100 g) vegetable shortening

1 cup (125 g) white rice flour

½ cup (65 g) corn, tapioca, or arrowroot starch

½ cup (50 g) powdered sugar (contains cornstarch, use corn-free recipe on page 103)

⅛ teaspoon (0.6 g) baking powder

⅛ teaspoon (0.75 g) salt

Lemon Filling:

½ cup (65 g) corn, tapioca, or arrowroot starch

1¼ cups (250 g) sugar

1 cup (235 ml) water

1½ cups (355 ml) lemon juice

1 teaspoon (1.7 g) lemon zest

1 cup fresh (130 g) raspberries, blueberries, or blackberries

1. Preheat oven to 350°F (180°C, or gas mark 4).

2. To make the crust: Combine all crust ingredients in a food processor and process until dough forms into a ball. Press crust into a 9 × 13-inch (23 × 33-cm) baking pan. Bake for 25 minutes. Let cool.

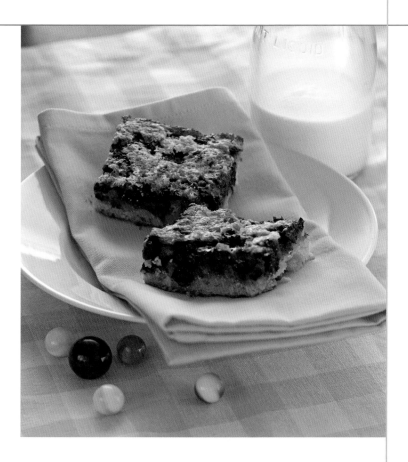

3. To make filling: Combine starch, sugar, water, lemon juice, and lemon zest in a saucepan. Over medium heat, bring to a gentle boil while stirring constantly. Lower the heat and cook for 1 minute, continuing to stir. Gently stir in berries. Pour lemon mixture over crust. Let cool and place in the refrigerator to chill.

4. Sift powdered sugar heavily over the top. Cut into bars.

Yield: 16 bars

Currant Hermits

It seems to me that toddlers always like these. You get a lot of fiber, iron, and nutrients in this little cookie.

½ cup (120 ml) olive oil

¾ cup (170 g) brown sugar

¼ cup (60 ml) molasses

1½ cups (190 g) brown rice flour

¼ cup (28 g) ground flax meal

1 teaspoon (2.3 g) cinnamon

½ teaspoon (2.3 g) baking soda

½ teaspoon (3 g) salt

½ teaspoon (1.1 g) ground nutmeg

¼ cup (60 ml) alternative milk beverages

1 cup (150 g) currants

1 cup (225 g) pumpkin or sunflower seeds

1. Preheat oven to 375°F (190°C, or gas mark 5).
2. In a mixer, cream together oil, brown sugar, and molasses. Add the flour, flax meal, cinnamon, baking soda, salt, and nutmeg. Slowly pour in the milk while mixing in the dry ingredients, scraping down the sides of the bowl.
3. Drop dough by rounded teaspoonfuls onto a greased baking sheet, spacing 1 inch (2.5 cm) apart.
4. Bake until lightly browned, about 10 minutes. Let them cool slightly and then remove to a cooling rack until completely cooled.

Yield: about 36 cookies

Oatmeal Cranberry Glazed Cookies

For a holiday flare, add 1 teaspoon (1.7 g) orange zest.

- 1 cup (200 g) vegetable shortening
- 1 tablespoon (15 ml) canola oil
- 1 teaspoon (5 ml) vanilla extract
- 1 cup (225 g) brown sugar
- 1½ cups (120 g) old-fashioned certified gluten-free oats
- 1 cup (125 g) white or brown rice flour
- ½ cup (56 g) flax meal
- 1 teaspoon (4.6 g) baking soda
- ½ teaspoon (3 g) salt
- 6 ounces (170 g) dried cranberries
- ½ cup (50 g) powdered sugar (contains cornstarch, use corn-free recipe on page 103)
- A few teaspoons alternative milk beverage

1. Preheat oven to 350°F (180°C, or gas mark 4).

2. In a mixer, cream together the shortening, oil, vanilla, and brown sugar. Mix in the certified gluten-free oats, flour, flax meal, baking soda, and salt. Stir in the cranberries. Drop by rounded teaspoonfuls onto a baking sheet. Bake for 10 minutes. Let cool completely on baking sheet.

3. While cookies are baking, mix together the powdered sugar and a little milk alternative to make a glaze for drizzling. With a spoon, drizzle powdered sugar glaze over each cooled cookie.

Yield: 24 cookies

Chewy Oatmeal Raisin Cookies

There is something about an oatmeal cookie that I love. This recipe is one of my favorites. With its high oatmeal content, it offers a lot of roughage for a cookie. I often have one mid-morning with a cup of tea.

1 cup (235 ml) natural maple syrup

¾ cup (170 g) vegetable shortening

1 teaspoon (5 ml) vanilla extract

3 cups (240 g) certified gluten-free oats

1 cup (125 g) white or brown rice flour or certified gluten-free oat flour

½ teaspoon (2.3 g) baking soda

¼ teaspoon (1.5 g) salt

1 teaspoon (2.3 g) cinnamon

1 cup (145 g) raisins

1. Preheat oven to 350°F (180°C, or gas mark 4).
2. In a mixer, cream together the syrup, shortening, and vanilla. Add in remaining ingredients except for raisins. Mix well. Stir in raisins by hand.
3. Using a medium-size cookie scoop, drop dough onto a baking sheet. Flatten each cookie slightly with your hand.
4. Bake for 10 minutes. For chewier cookies, remove before edges brown. Let cool on baking sheet and then remove with a spatula.

Yield: 36 cookies

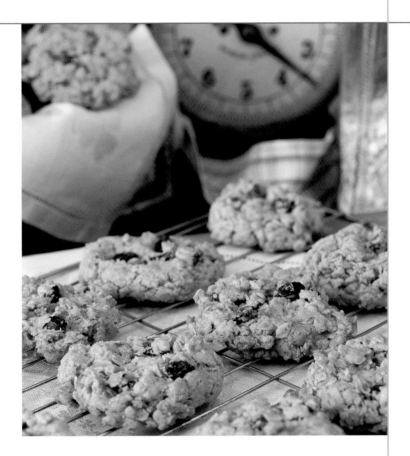

Cooking is a Family Affair

I call myself the weekend baker! It takes a few days a week to prepare foods like muffins, mini-quiches, and crackers and then freeze and package them to eat whenever you want. Once you get started, it is a breeze! I always look at my food preparation in a positive light, regardless of our allergies and my celiac disease. I feel truly blessed to know that my family is eating foods that I have prepared with love. They have no chemicals, are low sugar, and have no preservatives—just allergy-free goodness!

Healthy Cookie

These are surprisingly good little biscuit cookies. You may add a teaspoon of cinnamon or orange zest if desired.

1 cup (250 g) applesauce

¼ cup (55 g) brown sugar

¼ cup (50 g) white sugar

2½ cups (310 g) rice flour

1 teaspoon (6 g) salt

1 teaspoon (4.6 g) baking soda

1 teaspoon (4.6 g) baking powder

2 cups (350 g) raisins, dates, or other dried fruit

1. Preheat oven to 350°F (180°C, or gas mark 4).
2. In a mixer, cream together the applesauce and the sugars. Add the flour, salt, baking soda, and baking powder and blend well. Stir in the dried fruit.
3. Drop 2-inch (5-cm) mounds of dough onto a greased baking sheet. Bake for 8 minutes or until firm. Cool completely on the baking sheet. Store in a covered container.

Yield: 30 cookies

No Bake "Nutty" Bites

½ cup (130 g) sunflower butter

¼ cup (60 ml) brown rice syrup

1 cup (165 g) raisins

½ cup (87 g) allergy-safe semisweet chocolate chips (optional)

1. In a bowl, mix together the sunflower butter and brown rice syrup. Stir in raisins and chocolate chips.
2. Form into 2-inch (5-cm) balls. Place on a baking sheet lined with aluminum foil or nonstick parchment paper. Chill in the refrigerator.

Yield: 30 cookies

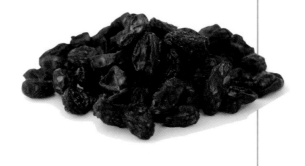

My Madeleines

Specialty Cookie Shapes

Specialty cookies get their distinct, well-defined shapes from special tools. French madeleines are baked in madeleine plaques; spicy Dutch speculaas are pressed into carved wooden molds; Swedish spritz cookies are formed into wreaths, ribbons, rosettes, and other shapes using a cookie press fitted with a decorative template; and German springerle are formed using a special carved rolling pin. The dough is stamped with the design, cut out, and then allowed to dry overnight to set the design before the cookies are baked. Try these fun shapes and use the opportunity to teach your children about other cultures at the same time!

Madeleines are little shell-shaped cookies that are dainty and buttery. My little Madeline likes to eat our version while we go shopping!

¼ cup (32 g) corn, tapioca, or arrowroot starch

1 cup (125 g) white rice flour

½ cup (120 ml) alternative milk beverage

2 teaspoons baking powder

½ teaspoon salt

¼ cup (60 ml) vegetable oil

1 cup (200 g) sugar

2 teaspoons lemon zest

1. Preheat oven to 375°F (190°C, or gas mark 5).
2. In a large bowl, combine all ingredients. Gently stir until you have a smooth batter.
3. Spoon dough into each shell of a well-greased Madeleine mold, filling to the top. Bake for 8 minutes, or until golden. Quickly remove from mold; you can use a butter knife to gently lift out. Let cool on a rack. Sprinkle with powdered sugar, if desired.

Yield: about 12 cookies

Oh Whee Ohs

For Cookie:

½ cup (100 g) vegetable shortening

1 cup (200 g) sugar

¾ cup (65 g) unsweetened cocoa powder

½ teaspoon (3 g) salt

½ cup (60 g) tapioca flour

2 cups (250 g) white or brown rice flour

¼ teaspoon baking powder

1 teaspoon baking soda

For Filling:

½ cup (100 g) vegetable shortening

2 cups (200 g) powdered sugar (contains corn starch, use corn-free recipe on page 103)

1 tablespoon (15 ml) vanilla

2 teaspoons (10 ml) alternative milk beverage or water

1. Preheat oven to 350°F (180°C, or gas mark 4).

2. To make the cookies: In a food processor, pulse together the shortening, ½ cup (120 ml) water, sugar, cocoa, and salt. Add flours, baking powder, and soda. Blend until dough forms a ball.

3. Take a 1-inch (2.5-cm) piece of dough and roll into a ball. Place 6 balls on a baking sheet lined with foil. Flatten evenly.

4. Bake for about 9 to 10 minutes or until the tops appear crackled. Let the cookies sit on the baking sheet for 2 minutes to cool slightly. The cookies should be firm like crackers. Once the cookies are the desired hardness, take a fork and make crisscrossing indentations on each. Carefully lift cookies off of the foil and let cool on a flat surface or refrigerate.

5. To make the filling: Place all filling ingredients into a clean food processor. Blend until smooth and thick, like butter. Frost the flat side of one chocolate cookie. Sandwich the flat side of another cookie over the frosting. Repeat.

Yield: about 25 sandwich cookies

Baker's Secret

The secret to perfect gluten-free cookies is to let them sit and cool as long as possible to prevent crumbling. For easy and inexpensive baking, line your baking sheets with aluminum foil! After removing cookies from the oven, let sit for 5 minutes. When cool to the touch, lift the corners of the foil up and gently lay on a flat surface to continue cooling. Simply re-line baking sheet and repeat. This also works well for brownies and cake.

Marshmallow Crunchy Bar Cut-Outs

Allergy-Safe Cereals

EnviroKidz cereals are available in many grocery stores. They offer kid-friendly cereals that cater to people with many kinds of food allergies: Amazon Frosted Flakes, Gorilla Munch, and Koala Krisp, to name a few. Look for Perky'o's allergy-friendly cereals too.

Take your average marshmallow/crisp rice cereal treat and jazz it up for fun! Use organic, gluten-free, whole-grain cereal.

7 cups (350 g) mini marshmallows

⅔ cup (170 g) vegetable shortening or oil

½ teaspoon (6 g) salt

5 cups (150 g) rice or corn cereal (rice, puffed cocoa crisps, or fruit crisps)

2 teaspoons (10 ml) vanilla extract

1 cup (200 g) candy pieces of your choice

1. In a large pot over low heat, melt the shortening, marshmallows, and salt. Stir in the cereal and the vanilla, making sure to coat each piece of cereal. Stir in candy pieces.

2. Line a baking sheet with waxed paper. Spread rice mixture onto waxed paper to the edges of the pan. Coat your hands with cooking spray and push down the mixture into an even, flat rectangle. Cool to room temperature.

3. Spray selected cookie cutters (like stars or teddy bears) with cooking oil and firmly cut out shapes from cooled cereal mixture. Remove with a spatula and place on a waxed paper-lined baking sheet. Decorate with frosting, melted chocolate, additional candy, or cookie sprinkles. Royal Icing (page 232) makes beautiful cookies. You can even insert a cookie stick in the side, wrap in plastic wrap, and give as a gift or a special treat.

Yield: 36 bars

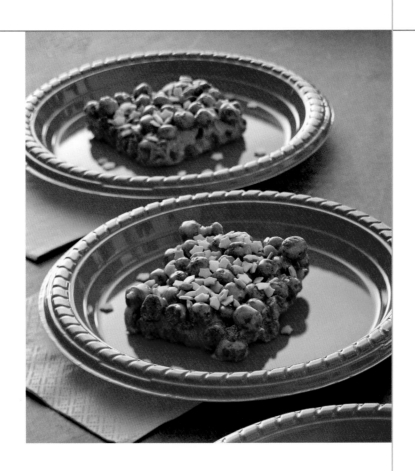

Frosted Brownies

This has long ranked #1 on the kids' Top 10 Treats list. I made sure this recipe would rank as high for everyone.

⅓ cup (80 ml) water

1 cup (200 g) sugar

½ cup (100 g) vegetable shortening

2 cups (350 g) allergy-safe semisweet chocolate chips, divided

¼ cup (245 g) applesauce

1 cup (125 g) white rice flour

½ teaspoon (2.3 g) baking powder

¼ teaspoon (1.5 g) salt

½ cup (120 ml) alternative milk beverage

1 cup (100 g) powdered sugar (contains cornstarch, use corn-free recipe on page 103)

1. Preheat oven to 350°F (180°C, or gas mark 4).

2. In a saucepan, combine the water, sugar, and shortening. Cook over medium heat, stirring constantly, until mixture comes to a boil. Remove from heat and stir in 1 cup (175 g) chocolate chips and applesauce. Stir until smooth and cool, about 4 minutes. Stir in the flour, baking powder, and salt. Pour into a greased 9-inch (23-cm) square baking pan. Bake for 30 minutes. Set aside to cool.

3. For frosting, in a small saucepan combine remaining 1 cup (175 g) chocolate chips and milk alternative and cook over low heat, stirring constantly. Remove from heat and stir in the powdered sugar. Cover and place in the refrigerator until thickened. Stir again and pour over brownies. Cover brownies and return to refrigerator until set, about 1 hour. Cut into squares.

Yield: 10 brownies

Double Chocolate Pound Cake

This works best as a pound cake or in a Bundt pan.

½ cup (125 g) unsweetened applesauce

2 tablespoons (30 ml) vegetable oil

1 cup (200 g) sugar

¼ teaspoon (1.5 g) salt

2 cups (350 g) allergy-safe semisweet chocolate chips, divided

1 teaspoon (5 ml) vanilla extract

⅓ cup (29 g) unsweetened cocoa

¼ cup (60 ml) water

1½ cups (185 g) white or brown rice flour

⅓ cup (42 g) tapioca flour

½ teaspoon (2.3 g) baking soda

1. Preheat oven to 325°F (170°C, or gas mark 3).

2. In a large saucepan, combine applesauce, oil, sugar, salt, 1 cup (175 g) chocolate chips, vanilla, cocoa, and water. Cook over low heat, stirring constantly, until chocolate chips are melted. Remove from heat.

3. Add flours and baking soda and mix with a wooden spoon until smooth. Quickly stir in remaining 1 cup (175 g) chocolate chips and pour batter into a greased 9 x 5 x 3-inch (23 x 12.5 x 7.5-cm) loaf pan. Bake for 1 hour and 35 minutes. Cool for 15 minutes. Run knife around edges and invert onto a cooling rack. Dust with powdered sugar, if desired.

Yield: 8 slices

Chocolate Cake

Cupcake Magic

Do the kids want Hostess Cupcakes? Try making this chocolate cake recipe into cupcakes and filling them with Vanilla Frosting (page 233). Simply cut out cylinders from the center of each cupcake and fill with frosting. Cut off the tips of the cylinders and place back over the frosting to cover. Frost the tops with chocolate frosting, then make zigzags across the top with the vanilla frosting. Yum!

This recipe is so versatile! It can make two 8-inch (20-cm) cakes, 24 cupcakes, or a 9-inch (22.5-cm) plate of brownies. You will be amazed at how tasty and easy to make this cake is.

½ cup (125 g) unsweetened applesauce

⅓ cup (80 ml) water

⅓ cup (80 ml) vegetable oil

1 tablespoon (15 ml) vanilla extract

¾ cup (65 g) unsweetened cocoa powder

1 cup (200 g) sugar

1⅓ cups (165 g) white rice flour

1/4 teaspoon (1.5 g) salt

1 teaspoon (4.6 g) baking powder

1. Preheat oven to 350°F (180°C, or gas mark 4).

2. In a mixer, beat the applesauce, water, oil, vanilla, cocoa, and sugar until smooth. Add the flour, salt, and baking powder and mix until well combined.

3. Pour batter into 2 greased 8-inch (20-cm) cake pans lined with nonstick parchment paper. Bake for 30 minutes or until firm in the middle. Let cool for 30 minutes before inverting onto a cooling rack and removing the parchment paper. Cool again until cake is at room temperature. Frost with desired frosting.

4. For cupcakes, fill 24 paper-lined muffin cups and bake for 15 minutes.

Yield: 12 slices

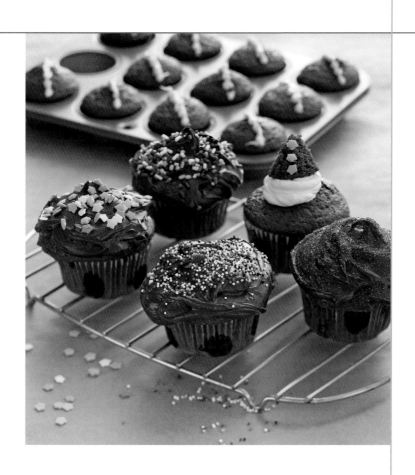

Creamsicle Cake

Frost with the Orange Vanilla Frosting (page 230).

Cupcakes for Everyone!
One of the hardest parts of being a kid with a wheat allergy is never getting to eat the cupcakes brought for all the birthdays in elementary schools. Even worse, perhaps, is when your birthday falls during the school year and you can't eat a cupcake, so you don't bring them. Now you can. Make up a batch of these for everyone! Your child will enjoy celebrating with all the other kids, and the other kids will love this wheat-free rendition of the old standby.

1 cup (235 ml) water

½ cup (120 ml) orange juice concentrate

1 cup (200 g) sugar

¼ cup (60 ml) vegetable oil

2 teaspoons (10 ml) vanilla extract

3 cups (375 g) white rice flour

1 tablespoon (13.8 g) baking powder

½ teaspoon (3 g) salt

1. Preheat oven to 350°F (180°C, or gas mark 4).
2. In a large bowl, combine all ingredients and mix until smooth. Pour batter into two 8-inch (20-cm) cake pans lined with nonstick parchment paper. Bake for 40 minutes or until firm in the center.
3. Let cool for 25 minutes and then invert onto a cooling rack. Peel off the parchment paper. Cool for an additional 20 minutes or until cake is room temperature. Frost as desired.
4. For cupcakes, fill 24 paper-lined muffin cups and bake for 15 minutes.

Yield: 12 slices

Pineapple Upside-Down Cake

2 tablespoons (30 ml) vegetable oil

½ cup (115 g) packed brown sugar

2 teaspoons (10 ml) water

1 can (15 ounces or 427 g) mini or regular pineapple rings, well drained, or 1 sliced fresh peach or apple

⅓ cup (80 ml) vegetable oil

⅔ cup (160 ml) alternative milk beverage or water

1 teaspoon (5 ml) vanilla extract

½ teaspoon (3 g) salt

1 cup (125 g) white or brown rice flour

½ cup (60 g) tapioca flour

1 cup (225 g) packed brown sugar

2 teaspoons (9.2 g) baking powder

1. Preheat oven to 350°F (180°C, or gas mark 4).

2. In a small saucepan heat the oil, brown sugar, and water for 1 minute or until smooth and caramel-like.

3. Line a 9-inch (23-cm) round cake pan with aluminum foil or non-stick parchment paper. Pour mixture into the lined pan. Arrange the drained pineapple rings or fruit over the mixture.

4. In a large bowl, mix together remaining ingredients until you have a smooth batter. Pour over pineapple rings. Bake for 45 minutes or until lightly golden and semi-firm in the center. Let cool.

5. Place a flat plate or cutting board directly over the baking pan. Flip over and remove baking pan.

Yield: 12 slices

Variation:
You may fill the holes of the pineapple rings with cherries, raisins, or sunflower seeds for extra décor.

Carrot Cake

These also make perfect cupcakes.

1 cup (200 g) sugar

¼ cup (60 ml) vegetable oil

½ cup (56 g) flax meal

1 teaspoon (5 ml) vanilla extract

2 cups (250 g) white or brown rice flour

2 teaspoons (9.2 g) baking powder

1 teaspoon (4.6 g) baking soda

1 teaspoon (2.3 g) cinnamon

1 teaspoon (1.8 g) ground ginger

2 cups (220 g) shredded carrots

1 cup (145 g) raisins or currants

1 can (8 ounces or 225 g) crushed pineapple, drained

1. Preheat oven to 350°F (180°C, or gas mark 4).

2. In a mixer, blend together the sugar, oil, flax, and vanilla. Add the flour, baking powder, baking soda, cinnamon, and ginger. Blend in the shredded carrots, raisins, and the crushed pineapple.

3. Pour batter into two 8-inch (20-cm) cake pans lined with nonstick parchment paper. Bake for 40 minutes or until firm in the center. Let cool for 25 minutes and then invert onto a cooling rack. Peel off the parchment paper. Cool for an additional 20 minutes or until cake is room temperature. Frost as desired.

4. For cupcakes, fill 24 paper-lined muffin cups and bake for 15 minutes.

Yield: 10 slices

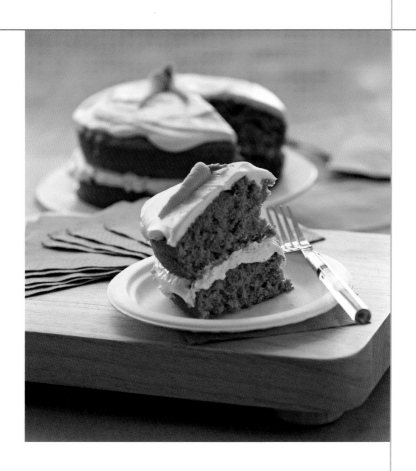

Gingerbread Cake

This delicious cake will impress your guests when you tell them it's allergy-friendly. Frost with Cinnamon Sweet Frosting (page 231) or Vanilla Frosting (page 233).

½ cup (100 g) vegetable shortening

2 tablespoons (30 g) brown sugar

1 cup (235 ml) unsulfured molasses

1 cup (235 ml) boiling water

2 cups (250 g) white or brown rice flour

¼ cup (30 g) tapioca flour

1 teaspoon (4.6 g) baking soda

½ teaspoon (3 g) salt

1 teaspoon (1.8 g) ground ginger

1 teaspoon (2.3 g) cinnamon

1. Preheat oven to 325°F (170°C, or gas mark 3).

2. In a mixer on low speed, mix shortening, brown sugar, molasses, and water. Add remaining ingredients and mix until smooth. Pour into a greased 9 × 13-inch (23 × 33-cm) baking pan or two 8-inch (20-cm) cake pans lined with nonstick parchment paper.

3. Bake for 50 minutes or until firm in the center. Let cool. Frost or dust with powdered sugar, if desired.

Yield: 16 slices

Celebration Torte Cake

For Cake:

½ cup (125 g) unsweetened applesauce

2 tablespoons (30 ml) vegetable oil

1 cup (200 g) superfine sugar

¼ teaspoon salt

1 cup (175 g) allergy-friendly semisweet chocolate chips

1 teaspoon (5 ml) vanilla extract

⅓ cup (29 g) unsweetened cocoa

¼ cup (60 ml) water

1½ cups (185 g) white or brown rice flour

⅓ cup (42 g) tapioca flour

½ teaspoon baking soda

For Topping:

¼ cup (50 g) vegetable shortening

1 teaspoon vanilla extract

2 cups (200 g) powdered sugar (contains corn starch, use corn-free recipe on page 82)

1 tablespoon (15 ml) water

Dash of salt

1 cup (110 g) fresh raspberries

1 cup (110 g) fresh strawberries, sliced

1/2 cup (70 g) fresh blueberries or blackberries

1. Preheat oven to 350°F (180°C, or gas mark 4).

2. To make the cake: In a large saucepan, combine first 8 ingredients (through water). Cook over low heat, stirring constantly, until chips are melted. Remove from heat. Stir in remaining cake ingredients. Pour into a greased 9-inch (23-cm) springform pan. Bake for 25 minutes or until slightly soft in the center and more firm around the edges. Let cool completely.

3. To make topping: Combine the first 5 ingredients (through salt) in a food processor and pulse until smooth. Spread over cooled cake. Layer berries over the top. Remove the rim of the springform pan, cut into wedges, and serve.

Yield: 12 slices

Math Made Fun!

Cooking can actually turn into a mathematics lesson. Whenever you use measuring cups, explain to your children the fractions of the whole. Your child will soon remember, for example, that four ½ cups make 1 whole cup.

Vanilla White Cake

This is a perfect birthday cake recipe. Frost with any desired frosting.

½ cup (100 g) vegetable shortening

1¾ cups (350 g) sugar

1½ cups (185 g) white rice flour

½ cup (60 g) tapioca flour

2 teaspoons (9.2 g) baking powder

½ teaspoon (3 g) salt

2 teaspoons (10 ml) vanilla extract

1⅓ cups (315 ml) alternative milk beverage or water

1. Preheat oven to 325°F (170°C, or gas mark 3).

2. In a mixer, beat the shortening and sugar. Add the flours, baking powder, and salt. Add the vanilla and slowly add the milk while the mixer is on low. Blend until smooth.

4. Pour into two 8-inch (20-cm) cake pans lined with nonstick parchment paper. Bake for 35 minutes. Let cool. Invert onto a cooling rack and gently peel off the parchment. Cool completely before frosting.

Yield: 12 slices

Birthday Star Cake

Having a birthday party? Try this Star Cake: Make the Vanilla White Cake in two 8-inch (20-cm) round cake pans, place one cake on a plate and top with a fruit filling, then layer the other cake on top. Frost with a white frosting. Make a recipe of Fun Cut-Outs dough (page 186). Using cookie cutters, cut dough into desired shapes (stars, baseballs and bats, soccer balls, ballet slippers, etc.). Bake and decorate the cookies. Press cookies into the frosting on the sides of the cake. Place a few cookies on top of the cake with the child's name on one cookie and "Happy Birthday" on another. Decorate borders with colored sugar or additional frosting. Decorate remaining cookies and send them home as gifts!

ALLERGY-PROOF RECIPES FOR KIDS

Wonder Cake

This cake is basically free of all allergens. It is, indeed, a wonder. It is perfectly full of taste and tenderness.

⅓ cup (115 g) honey

⅓ cup (115 g) molasses

6 tablespoons (90 ml) oil

1¾ cups (215 g) white or brown rice flour

Dash of salt

2 teaspoons (4.6 g) cinnamon

2 teaspoons (9.2 g) baking powder

½ teaspoon (23. g) baking soda

1 cup (235 ml) apple juice

1 small apple, chopped

1 small pear, chopped

½ cup (75 g) raisins

1. Preheat oven to 350°F (180°C, or gas mark 4).

2. In a mixer, blend the honey, molasses, and oil. Add the flour, salt, cinnamon, baking powder, and baking soda. On low speed, mix in the juice. Stir in the chopped apple, pear, and raisins.

3. Pour into a parchment-lined 8- or 9-inch (20- or 23-cm) cake pan. Bake for 45 minutes. Dust with powdered or raw sugar, if desired.

Yield: 12 slices

Low-sugar variation:
Omit honey and molasses.

Involve Your Kids in Cooking

Part of the fun of eating is cooking. Bring your children (assuming they are old enough) into the kitchen with you and teach them the culinary arts. I always include my little girls in the baking process. My toddler pulls the plastic containers and spoons from the cupboard, my preschooler likes to stir and scoop, and the oldest assists by preparing and putting away the ingredients. It is fun for the little helpers to have a few ingredients in their own bowls. Have them mimic you cooking or let them be the head chef. Make your own tradition in the kitchen, because, after all, home and hearth are the best of life, really!

Dream Berry Torte

If you miss cheesecake, try this frozen dessert in place of it. You can use practically any flavor of cookies for the crust to create your own delicious dessert. I like gingersnap, sugar cookie, chocolate, and even oatmeal raisin cookies for the crust.

3 cups (155 g) favorite safe homemade or store-bought cookies

¼ cup (50 g) sugar (optional)

6 tablespoons (90 ml) vegetable oil

1 pint (475 ml) Rice Dream ice cream or safe ice cream alternative, semi thawed

2 cups (340 g) fresh berries, rinsed and sliced or Lemon Raspberry Topping (page 220)

1. In a food processor, pulse cookies until you get a fine meal. You need enough to make about 1¼ cups (155 g) flour.
2. Pour sugar and oil into processor with cookie flour; pulse until the mixture is wet and combined. With your hands, mold dough together and press into a 9-inch (23-cm) pie plate or springform pan.
3. Bake in a 350-degree oven for about 10 minutes. Let cool completely
4. Stir ice cream and spread onto cookie crust. Place in freezer for about 30 minutes. Remove and top with berries or the Lemon Raspberry Topping. Let thaw for about 5 minutes. If using a springform pan, remove sides.

Yield: 10 slices

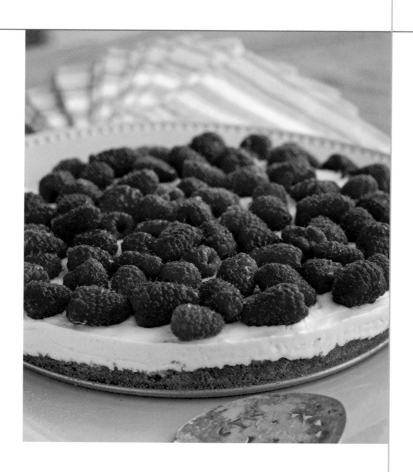

Lemon Raspberry Topping

Yummy Raspberries

Most people are familiar with the red variety of raspberries, but there are also black and white raspberries. Raspberries come from a rambling vine and prefer growing in cooler climates. Use fresh raspberries as soon as possible after purchasing as they tend to get moldy quickly. Kids love the sweet-tart taste and the way the juice stains their tongues!

This is a great sauce used in layers of cake or over ice cream. This low-sugar topping is a great way to sneak in the benefits of berries.

> 12 ounces (340 g) frozen raspberries (or blueberries), thawed
>
> ¼ cup (50 g) sugar or concentrated raspberry juice
>
> 2 tablespoons (30 ml) juice or water
>
> ¼ cup (30 g) corn, tapioca, or arrowroot starch
>
> 1 teaspoon (1.7 g) grated lemon peel

1. In a saucepan, combine the thawed raspberries and sugar or juice. Heat on low until raspberries begin to fall apart. Mix 2 tablespoons (30 ml) of juice or water with cornstarch.

2. Add mixture to raspberries and turn up the heat to medium, stirring constantly until mixture thickens. Stir in lemon peel and set aside to cool. Refrigerate leftovers, if there are any.

Yield: 2 cups (420 g)

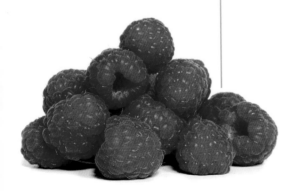

My Size Pies

Take your pick of which fabulous filling you want. These are the perfect treat for little hands. You can use your favorite tapioca-based fruit pie filling recipe in this too. Just cook it over the stovetop and pour into prebaked pie crusts.

1½ cups (355 ml) alternative milk beverage or water, divided

¼ cup (50 g) sugar

2 tablespoons (16 g) corn, tapioca, or arrowroot starch

2 teaspoons (10 ml) vanilla extract

1 recipe of any gluten-free pie crust or cookie crust dough, chilled

1. Preheat oven to 350°F (180°C, or gas mark 4).

2. In a medium saucepan combine the milk alternative, sugar, and cornstarch. Stir over medium heat until mixture comes to a boil. Remove from heat and stir in vanilla. Set aside.

3. Divide dough into 12 portions and roll into balls. Grease a muffin pan. Place a dough ball in each cup of the muffin pan. Use plastic wrap and added rice flour to keep dough from sticking to hands or wet your hands and pat in the dough to cover the bottom and sides of the muffin cup. Bake for 15 minutes.

4. Re-stir pudding mixture and fill each crust. Refrigerate for 2 hours, covered

Yield: 12 pies

Variation:

For chocolate pies, add 3/4 cup (135 g) allergy-safe semisweet chocolate chips to the milk mixture. For coconut pies, add 1 cup (70 g) shredded coconut to the milk mixture. For banana pies, add 1 thinly sliced banana to the milk mixture. For butterscotch, use brown sugar in place of sugar. For pudding cups, omit crust. For fruit pies, follow the pie directions on the back of a tapioca box to make a fruit filling.

Apple Rice Pudding

Variation:
For raisin pudding,
omit apples and add
1 cup (150 g) raisins.
For plain pudding,
omit apples, brown
sugar, and cinnamon.
Increase the vanilla by
2 teaspoons and add
1/4 cup (50 g) sugar. For
chocolate pudding, add
2/3 cup (120 g) allergy-
safe chocolate chips
in place of the apples.
Omit the cinnamon and
brown sugar. Stir until
the chocolate chips are
melted.

This is very rich, creamy, and delicious. Best of all, this is great whether served warm or cold.

3 cups (710 ml) alternative milk beverage, divided

2 cups (475 ml) water

1 cup (200 g) short-grain white rice

1 teaspoon (5 ml) vanilla extract

1 teaspoon (2.3 g) cinnamon

Pinch of salt

scant 1/2 cup (100 g) sugar

1 tablespoon (15 g) brown sugar

1 1/2 cups (225 g) finely chopped apples (about 2 apples)

1. In a medium saucepan, combine 2 cups (475 ml) milk, water, rice, vanilla, cinnamon, salt, and sugars. Cook at a gentle simmer over medium heat, stirring occasionally, for 20 minutes.

2. When most of the liquid has been absorbed, add in the apples. Cook 10 more minutes. Stir in the remaining 1 cup (235 ml) milk. Gradually stir into the rice mixture. Cook over medium heat, stirring constantly, until mixture boils and thickens, about 10 minutes. Spoon into individual bowls.

Yield: 6 servings

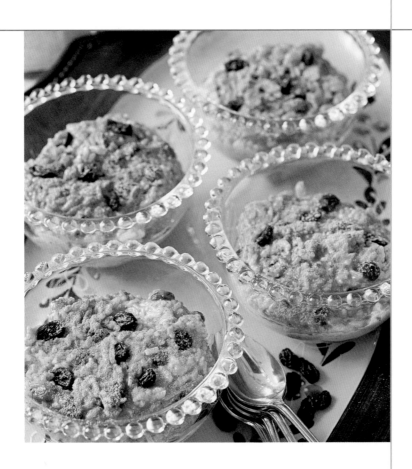

Low/No Sugar Baked Rice Pudding

The key to the sweetness here is to add nutmeg. This treat makes an excellent breakfast or dessert with whole grains and protein to start or end your day.

2 cups (475 ml) alternative milk beverage

1 tablespoon (8 g) corn, tapioca, or arrowroot starch

2 cups (330 g) white or brown short-grain rice, cooked

¼ cup (50 g) sugar or honey (optional)

2 teaspoons (3.4 g) lemon zest

¼ teaspoon (0.6 g) nutmeg

1 tablespoon (15 ml) lemon juice

½ cup (75 g) golden raisins

1. Preheat oven to 350°F (180°C, or gas mark 4).
2. In a small bowl, whisk together the milk and starch. In a large bowl, combine remaining ingredients. Pour milk mixture over rice mixture and stir well. Pour into an 8-inch (20-cm) greased glass round baking dish.
3. Bake for 45 minutes. Cool and serve warm or chill and serve cold.

Yield: 5 servings

The Perfect Pie Crust

I prefer this crust for all my fruit pies and my quiches. It is a good source of fiber, works well, and tastes great.

¾ cup (90 g) white rice flour

1½ cups (150 g) gluten-free oatmeal or rice bran

¼ teaspoon (1.5 g) salt

¼ cup (60 ml) oil

3 tablespoons (45 ml) honey or maple syrup

2 teaspoons (10 ml) water (optional)

1. In a food processor, combine the flour and certified gluten-free oats. Pulse until you have a blended flour. Add the remaining ingredients. Pulse until you have a firm dough that forms a ball. If mixture does not form into a ball, add water one teaspoon at a time and pulse until dough comes together.

2. Roll dough between two pieces of plastic wrap. Remove one piece of wrap and place dough (wrap-side up) on a pie plate. Pat dough firmly into pie plate. Remove remaining piece of wrap. Pour in desired filling and bake as usual.

3. To make crackers: Roll dough flat onto a baking sheet. Sprinkle with coarse salt. Prick several times with a fork. Bake at 350°F (180°C, or gas mark 4) for 8 minutes. Cut into squares.

Yield: 1 pie crust

Graham Cracker Push in Crust

Variation:
For a fruit tart, combine 8 ounces (230 g) dairy-free cream cheese or cream cheese alternative, 1 cup (100 g) powdered sugar, 1 teaspoon (10 ml) vanilla, and 1 tablespoon (15 ml) rice milk. Place all ingredients in food processor and process until smooth. Pour into pie shell. Layer a variety of sliced fruit and berries over cream cheese mixture. Refrigerate for 30 minutes and serve.

Be creative with this delicious sweet crust.

3 cups of broken-up Honey Graham Crackers (page 191)

¼ cup (50 g) sugar (optional)

6 tablespoons (85 g) vegetable oi

1. In a food processor, pulse graham crackers until you get a fine flour. You need enough crackers to make about 1¼ cup graham flour.

2. Pour sugar and oil into processor; pulse until the mixture is wet and combined. With your hands, mold dough together and push into a pie plate.

3. Follow the directions to desired dessert.

4. For a pudding pie: Use cream pudding filling from My Size Pies recipe (page 221) and fill pie shell.

Yield: 1 pie crust

Short Pastry Crust

This crust is very tasty and easy. Just pat it into whatever size pie pans you are using. This works well for sweet or savory fillings.

1 cup (125 g) white rice flour

1 cup (125 g) tapioca flour

½ cup (100 g) vegetable shortening

4 teaspoons (10.8 g) corn, tapioca, or arrowroot starch

1 teaspoon (6 g) salt

⅓ cup (80 ml) pure maple syrup, honey, or rice syrup

Dash of vinegar

1. Preheat oven to 350°F (180°C, or gas mark 4).
2. In a food processor, combine all of the ingredients. Pulse until it forms pea-sized pieces.
3. Roll dough into a ball. Place dough between 2 pieces of plastic wrap. Roll into a flat, round disk with a rolling pin. Invert into a pie crust tin and push to fit tin. Cut off edges.
4. Bake for 25 minutes or until lightly golden. Fill with desired fillings.

Yield: 1 pie shell

Rice Flour
Push-in Pie Crust

Chocolate Dessert Shells

To make chocolate bowls, turn a muffin pan over and coat the bottom of the cups with nonstick cooking spray. Drizzle melted allergy-safe semisweet chocolate over the cups to coat each cup well. Freeze for 15 minutes and then pop the chocolate bowls off the muffin pan. Fill with ice cream and serve immediately. You can place the ready-made ice cream-filled bowls in the freezer until ready to serve, if desired. These make great party desserts.

I changed the recipe a little from Bob's Red Mill. This is good for a sweet or savory dish.

1¼ cup (156 g) white rice flour

1 tablespoon (13 g) sugar

¼ teaspoon (1.5 g) sea salt

1 tablespoon (15 ml) cider vinegar or lemon juice

⅓ cup (70 g) vegetable shortening

½ cup (120 ml) milk or alternative

1. Preheat oven to 425°F (220°C, or gas mark 7).
2. Place all ingredients into a food processor. Pulse together until the mixture looks like crumbly dough. Press into a pie plate. Bake for 15 minutes. Cool and fill.

Yield: 1 pie shell

Candy Bar Chocolate Frosting

This delicious smooth frosting tops any cake and is good on a spoon too! For a quick treat, sandwich this frosting between two gluten-free graham crackers or cookies.

½ cup (100 g) vegetable shortening

3 cups (300 g) powdered sugar (contains cornstarch, use corn-free recipe on page 103)

⅔ cup (57 g) unsweetened cocoa powder

¼ cup (60 ml) water

2 teaspoons (10 ml) vanilla extract

1. Place all ingredients in a food processor and pulse until smooth.

Yield: enough for 1 cake

Easy Allergy-Friendly Decorations

Want to decorate your cakes, cookies, and cupcakes? Chocolate to the rescue! Melt your choice of allergy-safe chocolate chips, place in a resealable plastic bag with the tip cut off, and pipe out zigzags, letters, and stripes. Or melt together 6 ounces (170 g) of allergy-safe semisweet chocolate and 1 tablespoon (12.5 g) of shortening. Place in a bag and pipe out shapes like stars or hearts on a foil-lined baking sheet. Place in the freezer for 15 minutes, peel chocolate off foil, and stick on your cakes for a bakery-style dessert everyone will rave over.

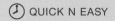

Orange Vanilla Frosting

My favorite of all the frostings! Unlike purchased frostings, this is flavored with real juice concentrate, not chemical flavorings.

½ cup (100 g) vegetable shortening

3 cups (300 g) powdered sugar (contains cornstarch, use corn-free recipe on page 103)

3 tablespoons (45 ml) frozen orange juice concentrate, thawed

¼ cup (60 ml) water

2 teaspoons (10 ml) vanilla extract

1. Place all ingredients in a food processor and pulse until smooth.

Yield: enough for 1 cake

Cinnamon Sweet Frosting

Spread this on spicy cakes like apple cake, carrot cake, or honey cake. Or microwave it a few seconds until soft and use as an icing on Bundt cakes or as a glaze on cookies.

½ cup (100 g) vegetable shortening

½ cup (110 g) brown sugar

3 cups (300 g) powdered sugar (contains cornstarch, use corn-free recipe on page 103)

½ teaspoon (1.2 g) ground cinnamon

½ teaspoon (0.9 g) ground ginger

1 teaspoon powdered vanilla

water

1. In a food processor, combine all ingredients and blend until smooth. Add water 1 teaspoon at a time until desired consistency is reached.

Yield: enough for 1 cake

Egg-Free Royal Icing

This dries quickly and has a beautiful, shiny appearance perfect for decorating cookies and detailed decorations on cakes.

> 2 cups (200 g) powdered sugar (contains cornstarch, use corn-free recipe on page 103)
>
> 2 teaspoons (10 ml) water
>
> 2 teaspoons (10 ml) rice syrup or honey
>
> ¼ teaspoon (1.3 g) vanilla extract
>
> assorted food coloring

1. In a mixer, combine all ingredients. Beat together until the consistency of glue.
2. You may thin with 1 to 3 teaspoons of rice syrup or water for drizzling over desserts or dipping cookies in. Or divide in portions and tint with different colors, if desired.

Yield: about 1 cup (180 g)

Vanilla Frosting

¼ cup (60 ml) water or alternative milk beverage

½ cup (100 g) vegetable shortening

4 cups (400 g) powdered sugar (contains cornstarch, use corn-free recipe on page 103)

4 teaspoons (20 ml) vanilla extract

1. In a mixer with a paddle attachment, whip the water or milk alternative and shortening together until fluffy. Add the sugar and vanilla; whip until smooth. Frost cookies, cupcakes, or 1 two-layer cake.

Yield: enough for 1 cake

Variation:
Add ¼ cup (45 g) melted allergy-safe semisweet chocolate after the sugar and vanilla. Or use 2 tablespoons (16 g) of cocoa. For a glaze, add 2 tablespoons (30 ml) of lemon juice. Use over a Bundt cake or for cookies.

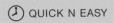

Honey Cream Frosting

This is not an overly sweet frosting, and it is great on any cake or muffin containing fruit. You can replace the honey with rice syrup, if desired.

½ cup (100 g) vegetable shortening

¼ cup (60 ml) firm honey (not runny)

2 cups (200 g) powdered sugar (contains cornstarch, use corn-free recipe on page 103)

Dash of cinnamon (optional)

1. In a mixer with the paddle attachment, beat shortening and honey on medium speed for 2 minutes or until fluffy. Add powdered sugar and cinnamon, if using, and blend until smooth. You can add a teaspoon of water to achieve desired spreading consistency.

Yield: enough for 1 cake

Homemade Marshmallows

1½ cups (355 ml) water, divided

4 envelopes unflavored gelatin

3 cups (600 g) sugar

1¼ cups (425 g) rice syrup

¼ teaspoon salt

2½ teaspoons (5 g) powdered vanilla

1 cup (120 g) powdered sugar (contains cornstarch,
   use corn-free recipe on page 103)

1. Pour ¾ cup (175 ml) water in the bowl of a mixer. Sprinkle with
   gelatin; let soften for 5 minutes.

2. Place the sugar, rice syrup, salt, and the remaining ¾ cup
   (175 ml) water in a saucepan and bring to a boil; let boil about
   4 minutes (a candy thermometer should register 240°F [115°C]).

3. With the mixer on low speed, carefully add hot syrup to the
   gelatin mixture, pouring in a long, thin stream. Increase speed to
   high and beat until stiff peaks form, about 28 minutes. Beat in the
   vanilla.

4. Pour mixture into a greased 9 × 13-inch (22.5 × 32.5-cm) glass
   baking dish. Let stand at room temperature for 5 hours or until
   firm. Sift powdered sugar onto baking sheet lined with foil. Invert
   pan onto baking sheet. Using an oiled knife, cut into desired size
   squares. Roll in powdered sugar.

Yield: 16 marshmallows

Cranberry Whip

I serve this for the holidays, but it is a quick, refreshing treat for anytime.

2 cups (190 g) fresh cranberries

one 15-ounce (420-g) can pineapple chunks or apricots, drained

½ cup (90 g) dried apricots

½ cup (125 g) applesauce

½ cup (50 g) powdered sugar (optional, contains cornstarch, use corn-free recipe on page 103)

1. In a food processor, blend the cranberries, pineapple, and dried apricots until chopped coarsely. Stir in the applesauce and powdered sugar and refrigerate for 1 hour. Serve as a sweet topping to holiday cakes. This is very delicious with your Thanksgiving turkey also!

Yield: 3 cups (560 grams)

Fancy Fruit

This is a fabulous dessert idea. Make it as simple or as fancy as you want. Try bringing this to a child's classroom party—it is a guaranteed hit!

15 strawberries

1 cup (175 g) allergy-safe chocolate, melted (milk, semisweet, and white chocolate work great)

Candy, colored sugar, or sprinkles

1. Wash and dry the strawberries. Keep the stems on.
2. Melt chocolate according to package directions. Pour into a heavy-duty resealable plastic bag. Cut a small tip off one side. Pipe zigzag strips of chocolate over each piece of fruit. Or pour melted chocolate into a bowl and dip each strawberry halfway in. Place on a waxed paper-lined baking sheet. Sprinkle with candy or sprinkles. You may use a variety of different chocolates to decorate with. Be creative! Refrigerate until ready to use.

Yield: 15 strawberries

Variation:
Fresh pineapple spears and apple slices are also good. Make sure they are washed and dried really well. Coat banana slices in chocolate and freeze them for a yummy frozen treat.

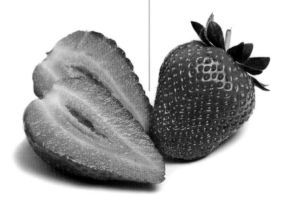

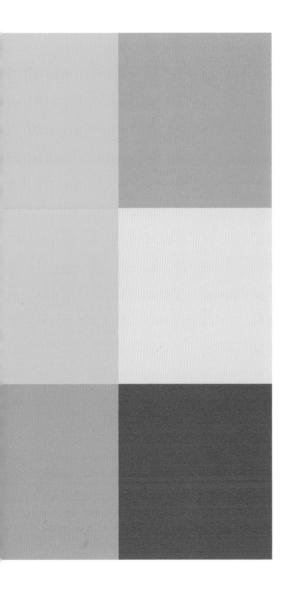

HELPFUL HINTS

Here are some helpful tips to keep kids feeling more included during parties and school activities. Most art materials like play dough and paints are made from potential irritants from dairy, peanut, or gluten. You can go online to www.nickelodeon.com for fun slime and dough ideas, just make sure to use the cornstarch-based recipes (you can substitute tapioca starch, if desired). Remember, just because your child has food restrictions does not mean she can't have a fun birthday party!

The Dream Princess Party

Celebrate your little princess in delicious style. Make a variety of hand-held snacks, including the following:

Fruit and Protein Dip (page 32) and fresh fruit slices

On the Trail Mix (page 36)

Sweet Rice Snacks (page 44)

Awesome Fluffy Lemon Blueberry Muffins—just make them mini (page 80)

Serve with lemonade or the Horchata Rice drink (page 24).

Barbie Doll Cake

Vanilla White Cake (page 216; double the recipe)

4 containers of gluten-free purchased vanilla frosting or Vanilla Frosting (page 233; quadruple the recipe)

1. Preheat oven to 325°F (170°C, or gas mark 3).

2. Prepare Vanilla White Cake according to directions and pour batter into two foil-lined Bundt pans.

3. Bake for 60 minutes or until the cake springs back at the center (this may require more time if you bake both cakes at once). Let cool for 20 minutes. Invert onto a cooling rack and peel off foil.

4. Turn one cake bottom-side up and push a Dixie cup into the bottom. Frost. Place the second cake bottom-side down on top of the frosted cake. Stand a new Barbie doll into the center of the cake. Lift her arms and tie up her hair. Frost her entire dress (the cake) and tint remaining frosting with desired colors. Then place this remaining, colored frosting in pastry bags or resealable plastic bags with the corners cut off and use that to decorate the cake. You may follow the pattern of a Princess Barbie box or consult a cake decorating book. Sprinkle Barbie with colored sugar or use sugared roses. Decorate a large marshmallow like a cute present and place in her hands.

Yield: 20–30 small slices

The Little Slugger's Party

For a fun boy's party, make a variety of yummy snacks including:

Spinach Dip with raw veggie dippers and assorted safe
crackers or chips (page 163)

Quick Savory Crackers (page 42)

Baked Potato Nachos (page 65)

Serve with Green Monster Power Smoothie (page 28).

Stars and Baseballs Cake

2 cakes of any flavor you desire

2 recipes of your choice frosting

1 recipe Fun Cut-Outs dough (page 186), or Sugar Cookie dough (page 184)

1. Prepare two cakes from a recipe of your liking, using 8- to 9-inch (20- to 30-cm) round cake pans. Cool for 20 minutes.

2. Place one cake down, frost, and then place the second cake on top. Frost the top and sides.

3. Roll out the Fun Cut-Outs or Sugar Cookie dough and use cookie cutters to make star, baseball, and bat shapes. Soccer balls and footballs work well too. Bake cookies and let cool. Tint vanilla frosting with colors like blue, red, green, and yellow and frost cookies as desired.

4. Within four hours of serving, place star cookies around sides of frosted cake. Place one baseball and one bat on top. Write the name of your child over the ball and write "Happy Birthday" underneath. Frost the border of the cake and sprinkle it with colored sugar. Serve additional cookies on the side.

Yield: 20–30 small slices

Fiesta Party Pleasers

Especially suitable to a buffet or large crowd, there is something here to appeal to almost anyone's needs.

Make one recipe of each:

Salsa Soup (page 152)

Tortilla-less Enchiladas (page 137)

Taco Salad (page 161)

Bean Salad (page 47)

Serve with chips and salsa. For a very large crowd, you can cut Mexican Pizzas (page 69) into single servings. For dessert, try the Chocolate Cake with Candy Bar Chocolate Frosting (pages 208 and 229) or Carrot Cupcakes with Cinnamon Sweet Frosting (pages 212 and 231).

Bunny Cake

Shredded coconut gives this cake the fluffy bunny appeal. If you are allergic to coconut, place a bag of allergy-safe semisweet chocolate chips into a food processor and pulse until you have chocolate flakes. Sprinkle the chocolate pieces over the cake to make a coconut-free bunny!

Carrot Cake (page 212)

2 cups (140 g) coconut

1 recipe Vanilla or Cinnamon Sweet Frosting (page 233 or 231)

2 strawberries

assorted candies and food coloring

1. Bake cake according to directions; remove from the oven and let cool completely.

2. Cut cake in half down the middle to make two semi-circles and frost the tops of each. Place one cake half on top of the other so their flat edges are facing you (it should look like a rainbow).

3. Frost entire cake and cover with coconut. Use candy to decorate the bunny face at one end of the "rainbow" and extra frosting and coconut to design ears and the bunny tail.

4. Cut two strawberries in half and place each half near the bottom, like bunny feet, with the large part of the strawberry in front and the small part pointing toward the tail. The cake should resemble a sitting bunny.

5. Use the same cake pattern and frost with primary colors to make a rainbow cake.

Yield: 15 small slices

Clay Dough

This dough dries nicely and is perfectly white. We paint our creations after they dry.

1 cup (125 g) white rice flour

1 cup (292 g) salt

¾ cup (180 ml) water

1. Mix all ingredients together in a bowl. Roll the dough into a firm ball. If the mixture is too crumbly, add additional water 1 teaspoon at a time.

2. Have children make snowmen, or use cookie cutters to make shapes.

3. Line a baking sheet with foil and let dry completely, for at least 1 day.

4. You can also bake the clay dough at 200°F (93°C) for about 30 minutes to harden and then paint as desired.

Flexible Play Dough

1½ cups (180 g) cornstarch

1/2 cup (60 g) rice flour

2 cups (470 ml) water

2 teaspoons (6 g) cream of tartar

1 cup (292 g) salt

1 tablespoon (15 ml) oil

1. Mix all ingredients in a saucepan and cook over medium heat, stirring constantly until the dough begins to solidify (this usually takes about 5 minutes).

2. Place in a large plastic bowl to cool. When dough is cool to the touch, divide into portions and place in a resealable plastic bag. Add desired amounts of food coloring to bag and seal. Have your child knead the bag until dough becomes evenly colored

3. Store, covered, in the refrigerator for about a month. Bring to room temperature before using.

Acknowledgments

I want to thank my publishing company, with a big thank you to Jill, Will, and John. I would also like to thank Julia for her outstanding editing. I want to acknowledge my children, Wendy, Allison, and Madeline, and thank them for their patience and understanding while mommy is running around frantic trying to finish all of her projects. I love you! I am so thankful for my grandparents, John and Jenny, for believing in me and helping me through so much over the years, without the two of you, being able to take on these projects, go back to school, and to be the kind of mommy that I inspire to be, would never have been a reality. My mom, Debbie, dad, Chip, and my brothers, Chris (see you soon) and Howie (Hi, Scarlet and Ashton)—I love you guys and appreciate what an awesome family we are! I would also like to thank my friend, Sarah, for always checking-in an making sure that I am all caught up on all of my projects! If any one understands what it's like to be a single mom of three, cheer coaching, going back to school (and having three kids in school), working, volunteering, keeping fit, and remaining sane, it's you Sarah! I do want to give a special thank you to my aunt Suzie for opening the door for new opportunities and for being not only my best friend, but also a great support. Yes, thank you to all of my special people who have supported and believed in me: Lynne Rominger, Jen Saunders, Beth Steinbock, Jen Childs, and Dr. Lee—thanks for always keeping my head on straight! I could not have done any of this without the encouragement from my grandma, Renee, I miss you. I would also like to thank the California Nutrition Network for the opportunity to share information on healthy families.

Leslie Hammond

Thank you Jennifer Basye Sander for bringing me in contact with Leslie and for being my friend and mentor. You are an amazingly talented, witty, and selfless woman who brings wisdom to my world. Thank you Leslie Hammond for your incredible recipes and passion for helping children; I've thoroughly enjoyed working with you and sharing everything from schooling ideas to home remedies to girl talk. Thank you to my parents and children—you are always so patient with all my work. Thank you "Dreamy" for providing some sweet respite for "Toula" amidst all my writing deadlines. You challenge me intellectually and make my knees weak. I feel blessed to have you as my friend. Thanks to the always-inspiring Derek Fromages; daily you brought levity to my life, and I doubt I could make it without the laughter you ignite. Thank you Christy Flis for your research, writing, and work on this book— what an amazing personal assistant you've been. A million "thank-yous" to Sabina Duncan. When I am frazzled and overwhelmed, you take the helm and lead me home. Thank you to everyone at Fair Winds. Finally, thank you, my Lord and Savior, Jesus Christ. I can do nothing without You.

Lynne Marie Rominger

About the Authors

Leslie Hammond is a culinary expert who focuses on allergies and allergy-free foods. She volunteers her time to educate the public and create awareness about alternative eating. She lives in Northern California

Lynne Marie Rominger has written more than one hundred feature articles for magazines, newspapers, and websites. She lives in Roseville, CA.

Index